The Fundamentals of Hospice Palliative Care

A Resource Guide for Health Care Providers

**Authors: Palliative Pain and Symptom Management
Consultation Program, Southwestern Ontario, Canada**

The Palliative Pain & Symptom Management Consultion Program of Southwestern Ontario, serving Erie St. Clair and the South West LHINs acknowledge the contributions of our colleagues in Hospice Palliative Care who have developed, refined and promoted hospice palliative care education programs throughout Southwestern Ontario. Because of their commitment, health care providers throughout Southwestern Ontario have a broader knowledge of Hospice Palliative Care and provide better end-of-life care.

Southwestern Ontario offers three distinct palliative care programs:

1. The Fundamentals of Hospice Palliative Care is an introductory education program based on foundational concepts from *A Model to Guide Hospice Palliative Care: Based on National Principles and Norms of Practice* (Ferris et al., 2002).

2. The Advanced Hospice Palliative Care Education program (AHPCE) is specifically designed to meet the learning aspirations and needs of support workers and volunteers.

3. The Comprehensive Advanced Palliative Care Education (CAPCE) for Registered Nurses and Registered Practical Nurses is again based on the National Model to Guide Hospice Palliative Care and builds on promoting issue identification in all domains, is supported by the foundational concepts and incorporates the steps of the Therapeutic Encounter.

Our goal is to provide learning opportunities for all formal care providers in Southwestern Ontario. In doing so we will raise the bar in providing best practices in end-of-life care to persons and families.

Support

Others providing support to the advancement of practices in the Southwest include:

- Lisa Malbrecht, Director, Complex Care Parkwood Hospital, St Joseph's Health Care, London, Ontario.

- Denise Eppel, Cabhru Solutions. Ontario.

- Diane Harris, Learning and Performance Consultant, Tillsonburg, Ontario.

- Megan Harris, Education Consultant, Milton, Ontario.

- Pat Hodgson, Logistics Management, Tillsonburg, Ontario.

- Julie Johnston, Coordinator, Palliative Pain & Symptom Management Consultation Program, Southwestern Ontario.

- Betty Tucker, Program Assistant, Palliative Pain & Symptom Management Consultation Program, Southwestern Ontario.

- Hospice Palliative Care Fundamentals Education Facilitators, Southwestern Ontario.

For information about the Southwestern Ontario Hospice Palliative Care Education Programs visit: www.palliativecareswo.ca

Acknowlegements

Focus

This Guide provides a written resource to the learners who actively participate in the Fundamentals of Hospice Palliative Care program. This highly interactive program includes 24 hours of in-class education and 6 hours of practical assignments.

The Fundamentals of Hospice Palliative Care is an introductory education program based on foundational concepts from *A Model to Guide Hospice Palliative Care: Based on National Principles and Norms of Practice* (Ferris et al., 2002).

This Resource Guide provides basic information, which is further developed through an interactive, case-based, learning-through-dialogue approach in the classroom.

Target learning group

Participants represent a wide variety of backgrounds, for example: volunteers, support workers, social workers, pharmacists, chaplains, physiotherapists, occupational therapists, registered practical nurses, registered nurses, physicians, and dietitians. This multidisciplinary group explores and supports each other's role and contributions to enhance the delivery of hospice palliative care.

Layout of Guide

This Resource Guide is divided into 12 chapters:

Chapters 1-2

- Introduce "A Model to Guide Hospice Palliative Care: Based on National Principles and Norms of Practice" (Ferris et al., 2002)

- Focus on the Model's foundational principles and concepts including basic definitions, values, and guiding principles

- Provide basic information regarding the domains of issues encountered by persons living with life threatening illness and strategies to address the identified issues

- Provide the information needed to develop basic skills and attitudes that will foster the therapeutic relationships that will change the experience of illness for those living with dying.

Chapters 3-11

These chapters deal with one or more of the domains in the Model to Guide Hospice Palliative Care and provide the learner with a range of practical strategies to influence care. Each chapter is sorted under a series of key headings to help the learner further understand and appreciate the importance of his or her role and contributions towards changing the experience of illness for the individual and family.

The content for chapters 3-11 is divided as follows:

1. Understanding the Fundamentals

2. Observing the Individual's Experience

3. Interacting with the Individual and Formal/Informal Caregivers

4. Providing Supportive Care Strategies

5. Working as a Team

6. Thriving in Hospice Palliative Care.

Chapter 12

This chapter provides definitions of commonly used terms.

> Please note: This Resource Guide is one part of a comprehensive learning and development strategy for the learners. The interactive, learning-through-dialogue, multimedia approach to the Fundamentals program is firmly based on adult learning concepts and best practices.

Performance Objectives

After full participation in the *Hospice Palliative Care Education; The Fundamentals* program, 6 months experience in his or her role, and with support from peers and managers, the expectation is that the learner will have the ability to enter into a therapeutic relationship with the person and family that will facilitate a change in the illness experience for the person and family.

The learner will:

1. Demonstrate sensitivity, understanding and respect for the individuality of the person, family and team/ caregivers involved in the illness experience, and seek an understanding of the domains of issues associated with illness and bereavement (i.e. disease management, physical, psychological, loss/grief, social and practical, end of life/death management, and spiritual)

2. Identify issues associated with illness and bereavement

3. Effectively communicate with the person, family and team

4. Recognize and report changes in any of the domains of issues associated with illness and bereavement

5. Provide palliative supportive care strategies

6. Actively contribute to the team approach to hospice palliative care

Table of Contents

Chapter One

Introduction to Dying, Death and Hospice Palliative Care

Disease Management

- Primary diagnosis, prognosis, evidence
- Secondary diagnosis (e.g. dementia, substance use)
- Co-morbidities (e.g. delirium, seizures)
- Adverse events (e.g. side effects)
- Allergies.

Physical

- Pain and other symptoms
- Level of consciousness, cognition
- Function, safety, aids (motor, senses, physiologic, sexual)
- Fluids, nutrition
- Wounds
- Habits.

Psychological

- Personality, strengths, behaviour, motivation
- Depression, anxiety
- Emotions
- Fears
- Control, dignity, independence
- Conflict, guilt, stress, coping responses
- Self-image.

Loss, Grief

- Loss
- Grief (e.g. acute, chronic, anticipatory)
- Bereavement planning
- Mourning.

Person and Family

- Demographics
- Culture
- Personal values, beliefs, practices and strengths
- Developmental stage, education, literacy
- Disabilities.

Social

- Cultural values, beliefs, practices
- Relationships, roles with family/friends, community
- Isolation, abandonment, reconciliation
- Safe environment
- Privacy, intimacy
- Routines, recreation, vacation
- Legal issues
- Family/caregiver protection
- Guardianship, custody issues.

End-of-Life Care/Death Management

- Life closure
- Gift giving
- Legacy creation
- Preparation for expected death
- Anticipation and management of physiological changes in the last hours of life
- Rites, rituals
- Pronouncement, certification
- Perideath care of family, handling of body
- Funerals, services.

Practical

- Activities of daily living (e.g. personal care, household activities)
- Dependents, pets
- Telephone access, transportation.

Spiritual

- Meaning, value
- Existential, transcendental
- Values, beliefs, practices, affiliations
- Spiritual advisors, rites, rituals
- Symbols, icons.

Ferris et al., 2002

Dying, Death and Hospice Palliative Care

Formal caregivers in hospice palliative care support persons with a life-limiting illness and their family members on a journey that will lead to death. It is critical that the formal caregivers have knowledge of dying and death. They must feel comfortable in its presence in order to create a space in which growth and healing of mind and spirit is possible.

Death is the inevitable outcome of being born and is a journey common to all living things. However, humans, by virtue of their ability to think and reason, are aware at both a conscious and an unconscious level of their eventual demise. The thought of death usually arouses a variety of anxieties and fears.

Death Anxiety

Firestone and Catlett (2009) define death anxiety as "a complex phenomenon that represents the blend of many different thought processes and emotions: the dread of death, the horror of physical and mental deterioration, the essential feeling of aloneness, the ultimate experience of separation anxiety, sadness about the eventual loss of self, and extremes of anger and despair about a situation over which we have no control".

Emotional Responses to Death Awareness:

(Firestone and Catlett 2009)

1. Terror and fear when considering the cessation of all consciousness at the moment of death. Personal reactions to this terror surrounding death may lead to angst related to:

- Aging
- Deterioration in health
- Thought of being on one's deathbed
- The omnipresent prospect of death throughout life.

2. Fears related to the dying process itself lead to:

- Avoidance of thinking about the process of dying
- Avoidance of association with the sick and dying since when confronted with deterioration in others we are confronted with our own mortality.

3. Fears related to imagining being on one's deathbed confront us with the immediacy of the inevitable along with:

- Fear of physical suffering
- Embarrassment at the possibility of losing control of physical functioning
- Frustration at lack of mobility
- Mortification at being totally dependent on others.

4. Fears related to death itself:

- Has been articulated using terms such as dread, angst, anxiety and terror
- Is fear of the unknown
- Is fear of the seeming randomness and impersonal manner in which death strikes
- Is related to the uncertainty regarding the time and place of our own disappearance from life; of never again seeing, hearing, tasting, smelling, feeling the sensation of pain or pleasure.

5. Fear of death as a final separation from loved ones

- Feelings of aloneness, isolation, and disconnection with each separation and farewell a reminder of the ultimate separation at death.

6. Anger and rage

- Fury that one will be deprived of everyone that one has come to love and cherish along with a sense of feeling cheated and robbed.

7. Shame and guilt

- Shame due to a sense of one's body being deficient
- Sense of guilt related to bringing children into a world where they will face suffering and loss can lead to parents to be over protective of their children
- Death guilt or survivor guilt has to do with self condemnation for having lived when others have died. e.g. survivors of the holocaust
- Existential guilt and regret from not having lived life to the fullest can lead to despair and alienation.

8. Sense of absurdity and meaninglessness of life

- Persistent feelings of despair and hopelessness can create a suicide risk.

9. Sadness

- Arises when one contemplates the death of oneself or of loved ones
- Anticipatory grief and anticipatory mourning often lends new meaning to life and enhances the ability to deal with distress.

10. Anguish and Guilt

- Deep worry and concern about the economic and psychological welfare of those one is leaving behind.

Neurotic emotional responses to the prospect of dying can lead to maladaptive behaviours that interfere with the ability to cope with life. Maladaptive behaviours include: obsessive compulsive disorder, hysteria, sadism, masochism, agoraphobia, panic disorder, as well as certain perversions and fetishes.

As hospice palliative care providers involved in the care of the sick and dying, we are called upon to look death in the face, not as an enemy, but as a natural and inevitable part of life. The extent to which palliative care team members have confronted their own death anxieties may affect their ability to understand the issues that the dying face as well as their ability to establish therapeutic relationships. We are called to embrace life in the face of death. Sharing feelings about death and dying with friends and colleagues and attempting to find meaning in our own existence can lead to death awareness on a conscious and an unconscious level and equip us to more thoughtfully approach our fellow human beings. Compassion and empathy grow in the conscious awareness that we all will die.

Historical Perspectives on Death

There are a number of ways in which to understand dying and death. Sociologist Tony Walter (1994) speaks of death in terms of 3 ideal types. The three ideal types are historical types with the traditional tending to give way to the modern, which in turn tends to give way to the neo-modern. The chart below has been adapted from Walter and indicates these changes over time. Western society's death culture is made up of these varied and conflicting elements. Different members of the same family may have contradicting ideas about death and how it should be approached.

Historical Comparative Analysis (Walter, 1994)

	1900-1950 (traditional)	1950-1980 (modern)	1980-present (neo-modern)
Bodily context	Death quick and frequent	Death hidden, institutionalized	Death prolonged, after long period of chronic illness
Social context	Community	Publicly managed/ privately felt	Private and public intertwined
Authority	Religion	Medicine	Self
Social death	Follows physical death	Precedes physical death	At physical death
Values	Respect for the deceased, for transition and for social mores	Dignity, privacy, independence, a fighting spirit	Personal growth, sharing autonomy, informed choice

An understanding of how different members within the family and within the team view death will enable the caregiver to interact with more sensitivity and compassion.

In the 19th century, death often occurred in the home. As was noted in the chart above, the 20th century saw significant change in the way people die. With the continual integration of new technologies into medical care, hopes for cure along with a more impersonal approach and a "never say die" attitude have evolved. (Meier, Isaacs and Hughes, 2010) As a result, for over half a century most people have died in an institutional setting, rather than at home nurtured by the family. Consequently, western society has become detached from the dying process, and many are no longer comfortable discussing the topic. There is a great deal of evidence to support the fact that western medicine contributes to the denial of death.

Hadid, (2009) explains that our attitudes toward death are influenced by our family, our peers, religion and culture, language, literature and the arts, and the media. What parents say and do informs a child's view of life and of the world. If dying and death is hidden, children tend to form their own potentially frightening ideas of death. If stoicism and non-discussion are the behaviours that the family promotes, children learn that emotions should not be displayed. As children grow, the peer group begins to have greater influence. Interactions with other families may expose the child to other ways of behaving in the presence of dying and death. Open discussion of the topic along with acknowledgement of the feelings and reactions when confronted with a situation involving dying and death can help the child to recognize that there are many ways of coping with death and there is no right or wrong way.

Religious training has an impact on the formation of attitudes toward death. Death may be the end of life on the physical plane and for some may carry with it the fear of final judgment. For others, death may be viewed as the end of suffering and the chance for a peaceful rest in a better place where all loved ones will join together in time. Death may also be a time of rest before entering into a new body and beginning life's journey again. Religious beliefs affect other end-of-life issues such as blood transfusions, artificial feeding and hydration, abortion, assisted suicide and euthanasia.

Culture has an impact on how one views dying and death and has a significant effect on conversations, choices, and the decision making process. In some cultures, the dying person is not to be told that he or she is dying.

Language around death is interesting. Euphemisms which are vague such as "lost" or "passed on" can distance the bereaved from the reality. Phrases such as "kicked the bucket" devalue and make light of death.

Literature and the arts offer many diverse ways of considering the themes of dying, death and bereavement. Music, opera, and novels, both fiction and nonfiction, offer us many thought provoking opportunities to contemplate our own attitudes around death and dying.

The news media informs us of death constantly with reports of death in war, assassinations, murder, accidents and catastrophic events. Over time, we can become desensitized to death.

In the movies, graphic scenes produce horror while death on TV is frequently sanitized and unrealistically quick. Exciting resuscitations insinuate that death can be avoided if we can just get to a hospital. Video games are graphic in their portrayals of death and characters simply come back to life in the click of a key.

Other factors affect the way we die. Our social network, our financial situation, our gender and our age will all have an effect on how we die. The extent to which family members and friends are available will affect the ability to die at home. Our financial status will determine the availability of interventions that lead to enhanced comfort e.g. complementary therapies such as massage therapy. The economic state of the family may also affect ones choices with regard to trials and alternative treatments. Women tend to outlive men and therefore women are more frequently widowed. Women will frequently lack a primary caregiver in the home when they experience deterioration in their health as they age.

Ageism also factors into how we die. Ageism, also called age discrimination is stereotyping of and discrimination against individuals or groups because of their age. It includes a set of beliefs, attitudes, norms, and values used to justify a way of looking at older people as weak, frail and disabled. The Canadian Network for the Prevention of Elder Abuse in their document "What is Ageism?" note that the term was coined in 1968 by Robert Neil Butler. Discrimination against seniors is patterned on sexism and racism. Ageism as a combination of three connected elements: prejudicial attitudes towards older people, old age, and the aging process; discriminatory practices against older people; and institutional practices and policies that perpetuate stereotypes about older people. Prejudices toward the elderly may affect their access to care and how vigorously they are treated throughout the illness trajectory. Ageism may affect the autonomy of elders when caregivers go to family members for decisions instead of getting consent for treatments from a capable elder.

Ageism in heath care could also be used to describe prejudice and discrimination against adolescents and children, including ignoring their ideas because they are too young, or assuming that they should behave in certain ways because of their age. Ageism affects the young in terms of mistaken caregiver beliefs that pain is not a serious consideration when dealing with infants or that children do not have the right to be involved in life and death decision making. It seems that the younger the person the greater the attempt to prolong life despite suffering. Masera and Spinetta (1999) as part of a working group who developed the 6th edition of guidelines for assistance to terminally ill children with cancer advocate that health care providers avoid a "ruthless obstinacy" approach; know when to move from cure-oriented therapy to palliative care.

Let's now take a look at a roadmap which depicts when and how our path of life with an anticipated future can suddenly change to an illness journey with an uncertain future. Entering this uncertain path can confront us with our mortality and stir up anxiety. For care providers, the roadmap can help us to recognize the path that a person in our care is travelling and how we might best support that person at different places on the roadmap. It also clearly demonstrates the need for professionals in all fields of medicine to have knowledge and skill in hospice palliative care or to know how those skills can be accessed.

NAVIGATING LIFE'S JOURNEY
A Roadmap to Support Decision Making

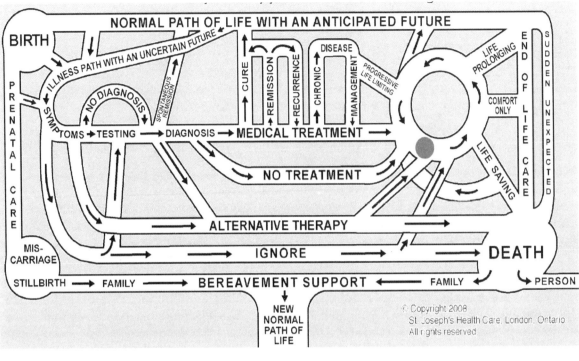

In the prenatal period on the left side of the map, families can be confronted with death through miscarriage, therapeutic abortion, or knowledge of a serious congenital anomaly in utero. Life can be snuffed out at birth or in the neonatal period from any number of complications. Through technologies such as ultrasound, disease can be detected and the fetus can be diverted from the normal path with an anticipated future onto the illness path even before birth. In order to support families through this crisis, there is a need for obstetrical and neonatal staff to have grounding in the art and science of hospice palliative care.

In infancy and childhood, symptoms can develop that put the child on the illness path. The child will go through testing, a diagnosis will hopefully be made and treatment instituted.

Treatment can lead to a cure or in the case of a progressive illness may keep the child on an illness path that impacts the rest of his or her life. If the disease is a progressive life limiting one, there may be a remission or the child may undergo ongoing treatment to manage the disease process. Pediatric staff with knowledge and skill in hospice palliative care can be of great support to families undergoing crisis. There is an emerging specialty within hospice palliative care related to provision of Pediatric Palliative Care.

In adolescence, acute illness, injury or chronic life limiting conditions can put the teen on the illness journey. Sudden death is always a possibility at any age but many a parent has spent sleepless nights hoping their teenager is not engaged in risky behavior. In this age group, suicide is also of great concern. The grief related to sudden death often requires the ongoing support of skilled bereavement counselors, but there is also need for emergency department staff to have skill in hospice palliative care since they are usually the first to attend to the distraught family.

At any age, people leave the path of life with an anticipated future and find themselves on the anxiety producing path of illness. While on this illness path, one experiences death anxiety to a greater or lesser degree. The person may be cured of acute illness and return to the normal path of life or they may find themselves on the road depicting the ongoing management of chronic illness or on the road of remission / recurrence.

At some point in the trajectory of a progressive life limiting illness the person comes to the circular road. Professionals need to recognize that the person is getting closer to death and support critical decision making related to goals of care. Goals of care will determine which road to take; the life saving road, the life prolonging road or the comfort road. Critical care staff and those in many specialties such as geriatrics, oncology, cardiology, nephrology, respirology, endocrinology and neurology need an awareness of the knowledge and skill developed in the field of palliative care in order to assist people in their decision making in these situations.

Death seldom comes without struggle and it is difficult for us to look death in the eye. We want to deny that it will come to us or those we love. Often when the diagnosis of a life-threatening illness comes, friends and family will encourage positive thinking and discourage any reflection about death. They may give advice about any number of treatments that could result in cure and will promote the adoption of a "fighting spirit". It is not easy for the person with the illness, or his or her family and friends, to face the inevitable. Being realistic about the situation can be equated with giving up on the part of the person or lack of compassion and concern on the part of the loved one or caregiver.

However, through open discussion about dying, individuals may find gentler and more meaningful ways to die. Delving into a subject that is sad, scary and largely taboo is difficult; however, witnessing it, talking about it, and learning about it can change the way we die. Field and Cassel in Meier, Isaacs, and Hughes (2010) are optimistic that people individually and together can take action to face death constructively and reduce suffering at the end of life.

Walking with those who live with dying is not easy but it is a privilege. The dying have many lessons to teach us. Some will teach us how to live with grace and dignity in the face of suffering. Others will amaze us with their wisdom. Still others will challenge us to remain calm in the face of anger and conflict. Their family caregivers can teach us about love and loyalty and commitment. Opportunity for personal and professional growth and development is ever present. One of the greatest lessons the dying teach us is to live every day to the fullest because life is fragile and precious.

Let's look at the history of the modern specialty designed to provide better care for those on that progressive life limiting illness path. The modern hospice palliative care movement that began in the 1970's is a promising alternative to the solely cure oriented and impersonal approach to health care. Hospice palliative care has ancient roots in the compassionate vision of those who were moved by the suffering and despair of dying people long before the advent of the modern health care system.

Dame Cicely Saunders, who trained first as a nurse then as a social worker and finally as a physician, was referred to at the time of her death in July 2005, as the founder of the modern hospice movement. She founded St. Christopher's Hospice in the United Kingdom in the mid 1960's to care for the dying. Balfour Mount, a Canadian physician, coined the term palliative care in 1975 because it was a term deemed acceptable in both English and French. The first hospital based Palliative Care Units in Canada opened the same year in Montreal at the Royal Victoria Hospital and in Winnipeg at St. Boniface Hospital. Both hospice and palliative care movements have flourished in Canada. Palliative care programs developed primarily within health care institutions while hospice care developed within the community primarily as volunteer programs.

To recognize both the convergence of hospice and palliative care into one movement and common norms of practice, the term "hospice palliative care" was adopted. While hospice palliative care is the nationally accepted term to describe care aimed at relieving suffering and improving quality of life, individual organizations may continue to use hospice, palliative care or another similarly acceptable term to describe their organization and the services they are providing.

Every hospice palliative care organization will have one of the following principal activities as its mandate:

- Direct care of persons and families

- Education

- Research

- Advocacy.

(Adapted from Ferris et al., 2002)

Today, the Province of Ontario is facing escalating health care costs; as a society, we are being challenged to set priorities. With new treatments and technology, people with life-limiting illnesses can be kept alive for many years. Management of chronic illness along with end-of-life care is a major concern for the health care system. There is also a growing realization that quality of life, as defined by the person with the illness, is as important a goal as prolonging life for its own sake. A shift is occurring. Health care professionals are being challenged to rethink the "never say die" attitude and to more actively engage persons and families in setting goals of care and making treatment decisions. Families are being required to participate to a greater degree in the care of their loved ones who are chronically ill and dying. Following years of advocacy, Compassionate Care Benefits are now a part of the Employment Insurance System in Canada.

The current vision of the Ministry of Health and Long Term Care in Ontario is one in which the majority of deaths will occur in the home with a combination of professional and family caregivers providing support for the dying person. Professional services are aimed at being proactive in identifying and addressing issues and preparing for crises so that visits to emergency departments and hospitalization can be avoided.

Reference List

Brayne, S. (2010). The D Word: Talking about Dying. Continuum International Publishing Group: London:

Canadian Network for the Prevention of Elder Abuse. *What is Ageism?* Retrieved from www.cnpea. ca/ageism February 2011

Ferris, F., Balfour, H.M., Bowen, K., Hardwick, M., Lamontagne,C., Lundy, M., Syme, A., West, P. (2002). *A model to guide hospice palliative care; Based on national principles and norms of practice.* Ottawa: Canadian Hospice Palliative Care Association.

Firestone, R., Catlett, J. (2009). *Beyond Death Anxiety.* New York; Springer Publishing Company, LLC.

Hadid, M. (2009). *The ultimate challenge: Coping with death, dying and bereavement.* Nelson Education: Toronto.

Masero, G., & Spinetta, J. (1999) *Guidelines for assistance to terminally ill children with cancer.* Retrieved from http://www.icccpo.org/articles/psychosocial/terminally_ill_children%20.html February 2011

Meier D.E., Isaacs S.L., & Hughes R.G., (eds). (2010). *Palliative Care: Transforming the Care of Serious Illness.* Wiley/Jossey-Bass: San Francisco.

Walter, T. (1994). *The revival of death.* New York: Routledge.

Chapter Two

Introduction to the Canadian Hospice Palliative Care Association's Model to Guide Hospice Palliative Care Based on Principles and Norms of Practice

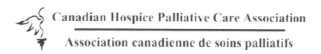

Canadian Hospice Palliative Care Association
Association canadienne de soins palliatifs

March 2002

The dying process is an inevitable part of the human experience. Feared by many of us, understood by fewer of us, the journey toward death is difficult for everyone. However, if the needs of a person who is dying are met, the journey can be a profound experience. Even in the midst of such an overwhelming situation, a person may find meaning and completeness to his or her life (Living Lessons, 2007).

The Fundamentals of Hospice Palliative Care is an introductory education program based on foundational concepts from *A Model to Guide Hospice Palliative Care: Based on National Principles and Norms of Practice* (Ferris et al., 2002). The program focuses on developing comfort around dying and death, familiarizing the formal caregivers with the issues encountered by persons living with life-threatening illness based on the Domains of Issues; Disease Management, Physical, Psychological, Spiritual, Social, Practical, End of Life Care/Death Management and Loss and Grief. Throughout the program, reference will be made to:

1. Understanding the fundamentals of each particular domain

2. Observing the individual's experience

3. Interacting with the individual and formal/informal caregivers

4. Providing supportive care strategies

5. Working as a team.

Learners in the program will become aware of the need to identify issues in each of the domains, the importance of communication and reporting observations while working together as a team to facilitate a positive change in the illness experience for those living with dying. This chapter introduces learners to The Model to Guide Hospice Palliative Care which was published in 2002 after over 10 years of consensus building among experts in hospice palliative care across Canada.

The Model to Guide Hospice Palliative Care (Ferris et al., 2002) provides direction to government, health care professionals, caregivers and volunteers as they attempt to develop services and standards to improve care throughout the illness trajectory.

Team members, depending on their specific responsibilities and accountabilities, play complementary and vitally important roles in facilitating a change in the illness experience for persons living with a life-threatening illness. Effective communication and effective group function are foundational to the process of providing care.

In 2005, the Ministry of Health and Long Term Care initiated a planning process to improve end-of-life care for the citizens of Ontario. A provincial advisory committee was struck to champion the project and to provide advice to the government as well as foster collaboration across the province. Each region was provided with funding to develop an End-of-Life Care Network to address system level issues. Local Community Care Access Centres were mandated the responsibility to develop a plan for integrated, interdisciplinary end-of-life service delivery that would ensure the following outcomes:

• Improved access to expertise in pain and symptom management

• Access to intervention for crises 24 hours a day and 7 days a week

• Enhanced services in the home to prevent emergency visits and hospitalization

• A coordinated point of entry

• Innovative use of technology.

Enhancement of collaboration and communication among various disciplines and across settings is happening as a result of Ontario's End-of-Life Care Strategy. Provincial and regional networks, as well as local service provider committees are addressing issues at the systems level as well as at the level of care delivery. The goal of these enhancements is to meet the needs of persons and families living with life-threatening illness by building and maintaining a system that supports formal caregivers to be proactive in identifying and addressing issues.

A paradigm shift is underway and hospitals are no longer to be seen as the most appropriate place to die. Deaths in hospitals will however continue as there are cases in which the person's symptoms cannot be managed in the home setting or there are not sufficient caregivers available to provide the necessary care. The hospital as the preferred site for death may be the choice of some individuals. Persons living with a life-threatening illness will, over the course of the illness, need to access services in various settings. Improvements are being made on an ongoing basis, to the collaboration and communication processes among various disciplines within and across settings. The goal of these improvements is to facilitate change in the person's experience, from one that may be inadequate or fragmented, to an experience that is proactive in identifying issues and truly meets the needs of the person and family.

Definition of Hospice Palliative Care

(Ferris et al., 2002)

Hospice palliative care:

- Aims to relieve suffering and improve the quality of living and dying

- Strives to help the person and his or her family to address issues, expectations, needs, hopes and fears; prepare for and manage self-determined life closure and the dying process; cope with loss and grief during illness and bereavement

- Aims to treat all active issues, prevent new issues from occurring and promote opportunities for meaningful experiences, personal and spiritual growth, and self actualization

- Is appropriate for any person and/or family living with, or at risk of developing, a life-threatening illness due to any diagnosis, with any prognosis, regardless of age, and at any time they have unmet expectations and/or needs, and are prepared to accept care

- May complement and enhance disease-modifying therapy or it may become the total focus of care

- Is most effectively delivered by an interdisciplinary team of healthcare providers who are both knowledgeable and skilled in all aspects of the caring process related to their discipline of practice.

Hospice palliative care is based on three foundational concepts:

1. Effective communication
2. Effective group function
3. The ability to facilitate change.

Foundational Concept 1: Effective Communication

Effective communication is critical to the process of providing palliative care.

Sources of difficulty in communication with those with progressive life limiting illness and those who are dying is discussed by Buckman in Emanuel and Librach (2007) under the following headings.

Social Denial of Death

- Lack of experience in the family

- High expectations of health and life

- Materialism: dying increases the penalty of death by being parted from material possessions

- Changing role of religion: not possible to assume that everyone shares the same idea about God or afterlife

- The person's fears of dying.

Factors that Originate in the Health Care Professional

- Sympathetic pain: discomfort is felt simply by being in the same room as someone going through the distress of facing death

- Fear of being blamed. When we are the bearers of bad news, often there is a notion that someone must be to blame when the person's condition deteriorates

- Fear of the untaught: many lack knowledge and skill in communicating with the dying

- Fear of eliciting a reaction: many have not been taught how to cope with reactions from persons and families

- Fear of saying "I don't know"

- Fear of expressing emotions: we are trained to hide and suppress emotions but when a patient is facing death, a professional who expresses no emotions is likely to be perceived as cold and insensitive

- Ambiguity of the phrase "I'm sorry": the phrase has two distinct meanings; a form of sympathy or a form of apology when accepting responsibility for an action. Rather than simply saying "I'm sorry", we should be more specific and say why we are sorry e.g."I'm sorry that happened to you"

- Our own fears of illness and death: our own issues can lead to avoidance or blocking of communication with the dying person.

    - Fear of the medical hierarchy: This fear can make it difficult to respond to a person's desire for information.

    Effective communication is aided by:

      - Using common terms, standard protocols and tools (See Chapter 10 for Definitions of Commonly Used Terms)

      - Sensitive sharing of important information

      - Education of all team members

Buckman in Emmanuel and Librach (2007) explains the CLASS Protocol for use when information is transmitted, when a dialogue is intended to centre on the person's feelings and emotions and the conversation is in itself a therapeutic action. The components of the **CLASS** protocol are listed below.

Context (or setting):

  Spacial Arrangements:
  - Ensure privacy
  - Move physical objects out of the line between you and the person
  - Ask that television, radio be turned off
  - Sit down
  - Maintain a distance (body buffer zone) of 2 to 3 feet
  - Ensure you are at or below the eye level of the person
  - When others are present, sit next to the person
  - Have tissues nearby.

  Body Language:
  - Move and talk in an unhurried manner
  - Sit comfortably with both feet on the floor, shoulders relaxed, and hands on the knees (neutral position).

  Eye Contact:
  - Maintain eye contact if the person is talking
  - Break eye contact if the person gets angry or begins to cry.

Touching the Person
- Can be of benefit as a show of support
- Be sensitive to the person's reaction; if the person is uncomfortable stop the contact
- Touching the hand or forearm is usually non-threatening
- Can be misinterpreted so requires self regulation.

Commencing the Interview
- Introduce yourself and explain what you do
- If shaking hands, shake the person's hand before others present at the interview.

Listening Skills:

Open Questions:
- Use questions that require more than a one word answer
- Open ended questions frequently start with "How", "What", "When"
- Avoid questions that start with "Why". Why questions seem to require justification for how you feel or what you did.

Silence:
- Wait for the person to stop talking before you start talking
- Silence may indicate emotions that are too intense to express in words
- Often means that the person is thinking or feeling something important
- A pause can enable the person to formulate the words
- A helpful way to break the silence is to say "What were you thinking about just then?"

Evident Hearing:
- nodding, smiling, using responses such as yes, Mmm, or "tell me more" demonstrate that you are listening.
- employ one or two of the person's key words from the person's last sentence in your response.
- reiterate to confirm that you have heard what was said.

Clarifying:
- When you have not understood what the person means, use phrases such as "I'm not sure what you meant when you said…" or "When you say …do you mean that …? "

Handling Time and Interruptions:
- Hold all calls if possible
- Turn off your pager
- If an interruption is necessary, express your regret and explain that you will resume the interview shortly
- For time constraints, explain that you have to leave and that you regret not having time to continue the conversation but that you will resume the conversation at a future time (provide a time).

Acknowledgement (and exploration) of Emotions

- an empathic response consists of 3 steps:

1. Identifying the emotion that the person is experiencing
2. Identifying the origin and root cause of the emotion
3. Responding in a way that expresses that you have made the connection between 1 and 2
   - If the person is expressing strong emotion, you must acknowledge the emotion or all further attempts at communication will fail.

Strategy for Management

- Determine what you believe to be the ideal plan
- Need a plan that the person will agree with and follow
- Determine the person's expectations of treatment, condition and outcome and summarize and clarify that understanding with the person
- Propose a strategy based on the ideal plan and what the person wants
- Constantly assess the person's response to the proposed plan, acknowledge emotions and continue to fashion a contractual agreement until you arrive at a plan that the person will buy into and will follow.

Summary

- This provides closure to the particular interview. If this will be a continuing relationship, emphasize that point.
- Cover the following three points:
  1. Reiterate the main points covered in the encounter
  2. Invite the person to ask questions
  3. Make an arrangement for the next interaction.

Buckman has another communication protocol using the acronym SPIKES. It is designed for difficult conversations particularly breaking bad news. That protocol is used in the CAPCE Program.

Team communication both verbal and written is very important. In order to avoid conflict that will impinge on the person's well-being and quality of life, the following chart outlines some communication strategies that support effective person to person interaction, family/ provider interaction and overall group function.

Communication Strategies to Support Effective Group Function

Common language	Care providers must share a common language and understanding of the definitions of the terms they use during the process of providing care. Caregivers must ensure that the person and family share that same understanding.
Standard approach to information sharing	Using a standard approach to communicate, listen and respond ensures that information is shared appropriately and promotes understanding. Sharing information with team members is appropriate if the information will assist in the care giving and understanding of the situation; however, respect the client by informing them of the need to share information.
Data collection	The collection of data that documents the person's and family's issues makes it easy to ensure that the appropriate team member engages in a therapeutic encounter that promotes desired outcomes thereby ensuring satisfaction. Document or relay information as per your agency's policy. Caregivers can assist the person and family by utilizing a combination of appropriate therapeutic interventions aimed at restoring the capacity to live as close to normal as possible.
Education	Education of the person, family and caregivers specific to their level of understanding, knowledge, skill, learning style and stress level will ensure that the person will enjoy the highest quality of life during this difficult time.
Good listening	The most vital role of the communicator is to be a good listener. We effectively communicate with others and build solid relationships when we take the time and energy to listen to what is being said and to hear the tone of the person's voice and see his or her physical actions.

Adapted from A Model to Guide Hospice Palliative Care (Ferris et al., 2002)

Foundational Concept 2: Effective Group Function

Every Hospice Palliative Care Team is comprised of various groups/disciplines:

- The person and family are core members of the team and come into the team with well established group leadership and dynamics. During illness, the group dynamics within a family, which may or may not have been effective in the past, may change dramatically.

- The primary and secondary hospice palliative care team consists of members of various disciplines involved in meeting the complex needs of the person and family. To be most effective this team requires leadership and consistent membership.

*See **Appendix A** for roles and responsibilities of various team members.*

- Group functioning depends to a great extent on an understanding of and respect for the various individuals who are responsible for supporting the person and family. Though there is a hierarchy in Health Care, palliative care seeks to overcome those attitudes and respect all members of the team as equal partners. (Alexis 2010)

The Model to Guide Hospice Palliative Care refers to Tuckman's (1965) stages of team development as a framework for understanding a palliative care team. In the provision of hospice palliative care, some members of the team (e.g. nurses, support workers, therapists) may remain stable while other members of the team (e.g. physicians) will change with each new case. Stein (2010) notes that stages are a "helpful framework for recognizing a team's behavioral patterns and they are most useful as a basis for team conversation, rather than boxing the team into a specific category. A team can maximize its productivity and facilitate a change in the illness experience of the person and family by understanding the functioning of the group. Just as human development is not always linear (think of the five-year old child who reverts to thumb-sucking when a new sibling is born), team development is not always a linear process. Having a way to identify and understand causes for changes in the team behaviours can help the team maximize its process and its productivity.

Stein (2010) has identified the feelings, the behaviours and the team tasks associated with each stage of team development. She has added an additional stage, termination, which in the case of the palliative care team would happen at the time of death. Though some of the same team members may become part of a new team forming around a new person and family, the composition of the team is ever changing.

Stage 1: Forming

Whenever a person's needs are identified as appropriate for hospice palliative care, a new team takes shape with the person and family at the center of the team.

Feelings	• Excited • Eager • High positive expectations • Anxiety about how they will fit in and whether they will measure up
Behaviours	• Lots of questions
Team Tasks	• Create a clear structure, goals, direction and roles • Build trust

Stage 2: Storming

The team begins to discover that they may not be able to meet all their expectations. Team members are attempting to see how the team will handle differences and conflict.

Feelings	• Frustration and anger • Express concerns about being unable to meet goals
Behaviours	• Less polite; frustration about constraints may be levelled at other team members, team leadership • Disagreement about goals, expectations, roles and responsibilities openly expressed • Team members may argue or become critical
Team Tasks	• Refocus on goals • Break larger goals into smaller achievable steps • Develop both task related skills, group process and conflict management skills • Redefine teams goals, roles, tasks

Stage 3: Norming

During the Norming stage of team development, team members begin to resolve the discrepancy they felt between their individual expectations and the reality of the team's experience. The team is successful in setting more flexible and inclusive norms and expectations.

Feelings	• An increased sense of comfort in expressing their "real" ideas and feelings • Feel an increasing acceptance of others on the team, recognizing that the variety of opinions and experiences makes the team stronger and its product richer. • Constructive criticism is both possible and welcomed. Members start to feel part of a team and can take pleasure from the increased group cohesion
Behaviours	• Members making a conscious effort to resolve problems and achieve group harmony • More frequent and more meaningful communication among team members and an increased willingness to share ideas or ask teammates for help • Refocus on established team ground rules and practices and return their focus to the team's tasks • Teams may begin to develop their own language (nicknames) or inside jokes
Team Tasks	• Members shift their energy to the team's goals • Show an increase in productivity, in both individual and collective work • An appropriate time for an evaluation of team processes and productivity

Stage 4: Performing

Feelings	• Satisfaction in the team's progress • Share insights into personal and group process • Aware of their own (and each other's) strengths and weaknesses • Attached to the team as something "greater than the sum of its parts" • Satisfaction in the team's effectiveness • Confidence in both individual abilities and those of their teammates
Behaviours	• Able to prevent or solve problems in the team's process or in the team's progress in meeting goals • A "can do" attitude is visible as are offers to assist one another • Roles on the team may have become more fluid, with members taking on various responsibilities as needed • Differences among members are appreciated and used to enhance the team's performance
Team Tasks	• Significant progress made toward meeting goals • Commitment to the team's mission is high • Competence of team members is high • Continued deepening of team member's knowledge and skills • Work to continuously improving team development • Accomplishments are measured and celebrated

Stage 5: Termination/Ending

Palliative Care Teams do come to an end, when death occurs. Their work with a specific family is ended. The nursing team may remain the same but there will be different partners in the next case; a different person and family at the centre, a different physician, a different group of PSWs and volunteers. While not part of Tuckman's original model, it is important for any team to pay attention to the end or termination process.

Feelings	• Members may carry a variety of feelings for the person who has died • Members may have concerns about the family members and their abilities to cope • Members may have some anxiety because of uncertainty about their future responsibilities • Sadness or a sense of loss about the death and separation from the family • A sense of deep satisfaction at the accomplishments of the team or a sense of frustration if the death did not go well • Individual members might feel all of these things at the same time, or may cycle through feelings of loss followed by feelings of satisfaction. Given these conflicting feelings, individual and team morale may rise or fall throughout the ending stage. It is highly likely that at any given moment individuals on the team will be experiencing different emotions about the death
Behaviours	• some team members may become less focussed on the team's tasks and their productivity may drop • alternatively, some team members may find focussing on the task at hand is an effective response to their sadness or sense of loss and their task productivity may increase

Team Tasks	• Need to acknowledge the upcoming transition and the variety of ways that individuals and the team may be feeling about the death
	• During this stage, the team should focus on three tasks:
	1. Completion of any deliverables and closure on any remaining team work
	2. Evaluation of the team's process and product, with a particular focus on identifying "lessons learned"
	3. Creating a closing celebration/ritual that:
	• Acknowledges the contributions of individuals
	• Acknowledges the accomplishments of the team
	• Formally ends this particular team's existence

Trust and respect among health providers is at the heart of interdisciplinary team work. Each discipline has its own set of knowledge and skills; based on education, training and experience. A collegial environment that supports all team members and listens respectfully to each person's observations, concerns and opinions enhances decision making, creativity and innovation. A commitment to teamwork and collaboration allows health professionals to learn from each other and gain an understanding of the competencies of their peers. (EICP Initiative 2006)

While working on a high-performing team may be a truly pleasurable and a growth experience, it is not the end of team development. There is still a need for the team to focus on both process and product, setting new goals as appropriate. Changes, such as members coming or going or large-scale changes in the external environment, can lead a team to cycle back to an earlier stage. If these changes - and their resulting behaviors - are recognized and addressed directly, teams may successfully remain in the Performing Stage indefinitely. (Stein 2010)

Groups that support the work of caregiver teams within the district, region and province include:

• A local committee with membership from various stakeholder organizations (e.g. hospitals, CCAC, Long Term Care Homes, Palliative Pain and Symptom Management Program) develops and supports the delivery of hospice palliative care services across settings.

• The End-of-Life Care Regional Network functions within each Local Health Integration Network (LHIN) to promote the system level coordination and integration necessary for seamless care delivery for the person and family.

• Provincial groups such as the Provincial End-of-Life Care Network, the Hospice Association of Ontario, the Ontario Palliative Care Association and other provincial bodies advocate on behalf of their members for broad system designs that will improve care delivery at the bedside and ultimately facilitate change in the illness experience for the person and family.

Foundational Concept 3: The Ability to Facilitate Change

This third foundational concept calls upon all care providers to become effective change agents in order to enable the person and family to live and die with the best quality of life. When symptoms of illness develop and particularly when a person is diagnosed with a life-threatening illness, the potential for a dramatic change in the way life is experienced exists. Such changes can be perceived as a threat to a person's capacity for meaningful and valuable experiences (Ferris et al 2002). The choices that each person makes will ultimately affect how the illness is experienced.

Change agents are individuals with knowledge, skills and tools. Effective change agents identify issues, gain an understanding of the effects of those issues, determine goals and identify possible solutions (Miller 2010). Effectiveness as a change agent is a combination of competence and confidence. For palliative care practitioners who desire to be effective change agents, education and training, practice opportunities, feedback and reflection and a support system are all required. Complementing the competencies identified above, superb communications ability with all members of the team is essential.

As change agents, the health care team members use their knowledge and skills to address all the identified issues. This may involve using logical arguments, facts, and success stories to overcome obstacles for the person and family e.g. fear of pain medications. The more expertise the team member is perceived to have, the more chance there is to be successful in changing attitudes and behaviours. (McShane 2008) Each team's effectiveness is based on the commitment to reflection and on-going evaluation of the team's accomplishments in terms of meeting the goals of the person and family.

The stages of team development can be applied to nursing teams, secondary level hospice palliative care teams, teams of volunteers/PSWs and other teams.

However, we always have to remember that the person him or herself is ultimately responsible for the decisions that will contribute to how the illness is experienced.

Palliative care providers are responsible for ensuring that their practice meets standards and that they constantly aspire to become increasingly competent in their role. Knowledge changes with new research, attitudes change with new learning, skills and behaviours change in response to new attitudes and knowledge. Change agents are needed at every level. Each member of the caregiver team, at all levels, is required to be open and adaptable. Every person on the team has the role of a change agent. At the bedside, the expertise of knowledgeable and skilled caregivers can be applied to identifying and responding to the multiple issues associated with the illness; and at the system level, identifying issues and gaps and working collaboratively with all stakeholders, leads to enhanced service delivery.

Guiding Principles of Palliative Care

(Ferris et al., 2002)

Person and Family Focused	• The person and family are always treated as a unit in a manner that is sensitive to the individual values and beliefs of the person and his or her family.
High Quality	• Activities are guided by these ethical principles: autonomy, beneficence, non-maleficence, justice, truth-telling and confidentiality, as well as nationally accepted standards of practice and norms of practice, and standards of professional conduct for each discipline, policies and procedures based on best practice, data collection and documentation guidelines that are based on validated measurement tools.

Safe and Effective	• Palliative care is conducted in a manner that is collaborative, ensures confidentiality, privacy, safety, continuity and accountability, is without coercion, discrimination, harassment or prejudice, aims to minimize unnecessary duplication and repetition and complies with laws, regulations and policies in effect within the jurisdiction, host and hospice palliative care organizations.
Accessible	• Each person and his or her family have equal access to hospice palliative care services wherever they live (at home, or within a reasonable distance from their home) in a timely manner.
Adequately Resourced	• The financial, human, information, physical and community resources are sufficient to sustain the organization's activities, and it's strategic and business plans.
Collaborative	• Each community's needs for hospice palliative care are assessed and addressed through the collaborative efforts of available organizations and services in partnership.
Knowledge-based	• Ongoing education of the person, his or her family or caregivers, staff and stakeholders is integral to the provision and advancement of quality hospice palliative care.
Advocacy-based	• Regular interaction with legislators, regulators, policy makers, healthcare funders, other hospice palliative care providers, professional societies and associations, and the public is essential to increase awareness about, and develop hospice palliative care activities and the resources that support them. All advocacy is based on *A Model to Guide Hospice Palliative Care* (Ferris et al., 2002).
Research-based	• The development, dissemination, and integration of new knowledge are critical to the advancement of quality hospice palliative care. Where possible, all activities are based on the best available evidence.

Role of Hospice Palliative Care during Illness

The figure below, adapted from *A Model to Guide Hospice Palliative Care* (Ferris et al., 2002), depicts the journey that a person takes; from the point that a life-threatening illness becomes a concern, through diagnostic procedures to confirmation of the diagnosis, to attempts to cure the disease, treat the symptoms and prolong life.

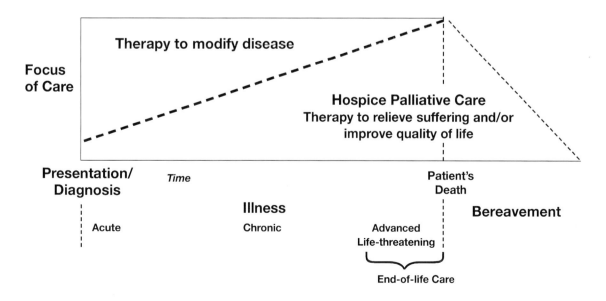

At some point, death occurs for the person with the illness and others are left to grieve the loss. Along this journey or illness trajectory, the person and family have needs that are best met by a combination of interventions aimed at treating the disease, managing the symptoms and providing support for the whole person, body, mind and spirit.

Interventions aimed at cure may be most important at the beginning of the journey, but the person will also have needs for information and support that cannot be ignored. As the person gets closer to the end of life, quality of life and the need for comfort and care may take precedence.

The diagram speaks to the balance that can be achieved throughout the journey. It is not necessary to forgo comfort if one wants to have life-prolonging therapies. Nor do all efforts to prolong life stop when the person is receiving palliative care. Hospice palliative care interventions should not be introduced days or hours before death but early in the journey. Since the family is the unit of care, support is extended into the bereavement period.

Types of Care

Despite the fact that a person may want to die at home, he or she may at times have needs that can best be met within different settings.

As an individual travels on the journey towards death, an understanding of the various settings where care can be provided enables formal caregivers to advocate on behalf of the person and family. It is important for caregivers to have knowledge of the available alternatives in the event that needs cannot be met within the home environment. Not every community will have access to every type of care.

Types of Care	Settings of Care
1. Acute care: for issues that require time-limited attention	• Acute care hospitals: including emergency rooms, intensive care units as well as on medical, surgical, obstetrics, pediatric, geriatric, and rehabilitation units • Offices or clinics
2. Chronic care: for issues that require continuous support and/or skilled nursing care	• Individual homes: including single family dwellings, apartments, retirement homes, boarding houses, group homes, correctional facilities, on the street • Complex continuing care • Palliative care units in hospitals or long term care homes • Free standing residential hospices • Long term care homes
3. Respite care: when caregivers become fatigued and require a break or a vacation	• Day programs • Individual homes
4. End-of-life care: when issues and the need for care can rise considerably particularly in the last days	• All settings
5. Bereavement care: for those who survive the person's death	• All settings

Potential Journey of a Person with Progressive Life Limiting Illness through Various Settings of Care

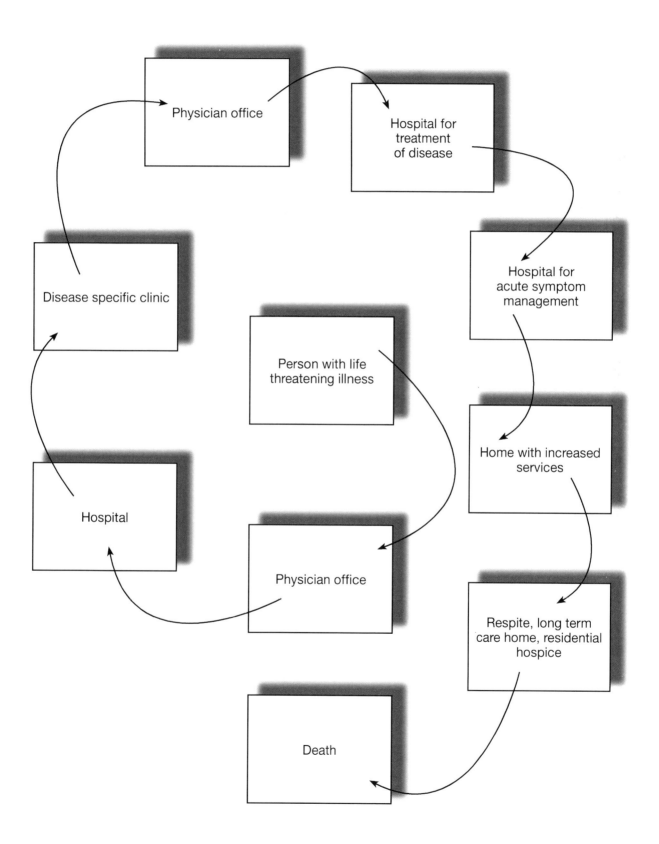

Service Delivery Models

Each dying person and family will have unique issues and needs. Primary care health care providers have always cared for the dying as part of their role and in many instances are capable of meeting the needs of the person and family. There are, however, situations when more specialized knowledge and skill would be of benefit to the person and family.

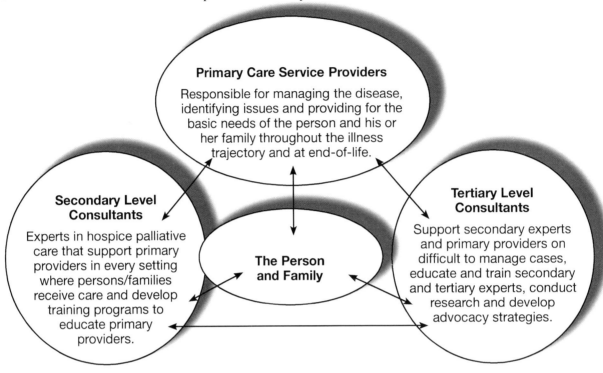

This diagram, adapted from *A Model to Guide Hospice Palliative Care* (Ferris et al., 2002), acknowledges the role of primary caregivers as well as secondary and tertiary level experts.

Hospice palliative care is a recognized specialty within health care. It is difficult for the generalist practitioner to remain current in every field. One of the roles of a secondary level consultant is to keep abreast of new research findings and best practice guidelines that can affect outcomes and share that information with primary providers. Mentoring and coaching is another important aspect of the secondary level expert's role.

Ideally, a system is developed to ensure timely access to secondary and tertiary experts who are available to support primary providers in their care of persons living with life-threatening illness. Secondary Level Consultants offers consultation that may include:

- Consultation that is one time with no follow-up by experts
- Consultation which is ongoing and support by experts with overall responsibility held by primary providers
- Consultation followed by experts assuming overall responsibility and primary providers maintaining a supporting role
- Consultation followed by assumption of care by experts with no primary providers involved in care.

Effective pain and symptom management is vital. If a person is physically comfortable and pain and other symptoms are managed well, he or she will be better able to focus on the equally important issues of mind, heart, and spirit. Awareness of community resources will help primary providers advocate on behalf of persons regarding specific needs (Living Lessons, 2007).

The Model to Guide Hospice Palliative Care based on National Principles and Norms of Practice has two very important concepts that are the underpinning for many education programs developed in Canada. Those concepts are the Domains of Issues and the Process of Providing Care. Those two concepts together are the basis for the Square of Care.

Domains of Issues
(Ferris et al., 2002)

Living with a life-threatening illness impacts a person and his or her family in all aspects of their lives. The issues are complex and multiple and can be categorized under the following headings or domains. Whenever an issue is identified in any domain, it needs to be addressed.

Disease Management
- Primary diagnosis, prognosis, evidence
- Secondary diagnosis (e.g. dementia, substance use)
- Co-morbidities (e.g. delirium, seizures)
- Adverse events (e.g. side effects)
- Allergies

Physical
- Pain and other symptoms
- Level of consciousness, cognition
- Function, safety, aids (motor, senses, physiologic, sexual)
- Fluids, nutrition
- Wounds
- Habits

Psychological
- Personality, strengths, behaviour, motivation
- Depression, anxiety
- Emotions
- Fears
- Control, dignity, independence
- Conflict, guilt, stress, coping responses
- Self-image

Loss, Grief
- Loss
- Grief (e.g. acute, chronic, anticipatory)
- Bereavement planning
- Mourning

Person and Family
- Demographics
- Culture
- Personal values, beliefs, practices and strengths
- Developmental stage, education, literacy
- Disabilities

Social
- Cultural values, beliefs, practices
- Relationships, roles with family/friends, community
- Isolation, abandonment, reconciliation
- Safe environment
- Privacy, intimacy
- Routines, recreation, vacation
- Legal issues
- Family/caregiver protection
- Guardianship, custody issues

End-of-Life Care/Death Management
- Life closure
- Gift giving
- Legacy creation
- Preparation for expected death
- Anticipation and management of physiological changes in the last hours of life
- Rites, rituals
- Pronouncement, certification
- Perideath care of family, handling of body
- Funerals, services

Practical
- Activities of daily living (e.g. personal care, household activities)
- Dependents, pets
- Telephone access, transportation

Spiritual
- Meaning, value
- Existential, transcendental
- Values, beliefs, practices, affiliations
- Spiritual advisors, rites, rituals
- Symbols, icons

Square of Care

In the 21st century, people are living with illness much longer than ever before. Today, they must deal with many complex questions: How can they get relief from their symptoms? How can they carry on life as they have known it? How will the illness affect their roles and relationships? How can they restore or maintain their capacity for meaningful and valuable experiences that give quality to their lives? What can be done to positively change the illness experience?

The Model outlines the Square of Care to order to provide a conceptualization of a process that can guide caregivers in establishing therapeutic relationships and ensuring that all issues are identified and addressed to the satisfaction of all concerned. Just as a builder's square ensures that a structure is built on a solid foundation, this square of care assists us in ensuring that our care giving is based on a solid foundation. This resource guide, The Fundamentals of Hospice Palliative Care focuses primarily on the domains of issues noted on the vertical axis of the diagram as well as the foundational concepts of effective communication, effective group function and the ability to facilitate change. The process of providing care noted along the horizontal axis is featured in the Comprehensive Advanced Palliative Care Education (CAPCE) course for nurses.

Square of Care
(Ferris et al., 2002)

Common Issues	Assessment	Information –Sharing	Decision-Making	Care Planning	Care Delivery	Confirmation
Disease Management						
Physical						
Psychological						
Social						
Spiritual						
Practical						
End of life/ Death Management						
Loss, Grief						

Reference List

Alexis, R. 2010 Hierarchy of Medical Professionals Retrieved from http://www.ehow.com/about_6517804_hierarchy-medical-professions.html#ixzz1CSxnDoWR

Berkeley Developmental Resources. *What is the change agent role?* Retrived January 2011 from www.bdrconsultants.com/agent_role.pdf

EICP Initaitve. 2006 The *Principles and Framework for Interdisciplinary Collaboration in Primary Health Care* Retrieved January 2011 from www.caslpa.ca/PDF/EICP_Principles_and_Framework_final.pdf

Ferris, F.D., Balfour, H.M., Bowen, K., Farley, J., Hardwick, M., Lamontagne, C., Lundy, M., Syme, A., & West, P. (2002). *A model to guide hospice palliative care; Based on national principles and norms of practice.* Ottawa: Canadian Hospice Palliative Care Association.

Grey Bruce Palliative Care Committee in collaboration with local service providers. *Palliative Care Team Member Roles* (revised 2011) In Grey Bruce Palliative Care Manual (1999)

Living Lessons. (2007). *Hospice Palliative Care Fact Sheet.* Retrieved January 2011 from http://www.living-lessons.org/main/a4.1.2.fact.sheet.asp.

McShane, L. (2008) Canadian Organizational Behaviour. Toronto: McGraw Hill Ryerson, Miller, K. (2008). *The change agent's guide to radical improvement.* ASQ. Milwaukee: Quality Press.

Stein, J. (2010). Working on Teams. Retrieved January 2011 from http://web.mit.edu/hr/oed/learn/teams/art_stages.html

Tuckman, B. (1965). Development sequence in small groups. *Psychological Bulletin.* 63: 384-399.

Appendix A: Palliative Care Team Member Roles

The roles of the following palliative care team members are defined below
(adapted in 2011 from Grey Bruce Palliative Care Manual, 1999):

1. Case Manager

2. Clergy/Pastor

3. Hospice Palliative Care Volunteers

4. Nurse, Primary Nurse and Expert Consultant

5. Occupational Therapist

6. Personal Support Worker or Health Care Aide

7. Pharmacist

8. Physician: Family Physician, Palliative Care Physician

9. Physician Assistant

10. Physiotherapist

11. Recreation Therapist

12. Registered Dietician

13. Respiratory Therapist

14. Social Worker

15. Speech-Language Pathologist

Individuals from various disciplines may be members of Primary Teams within an organization, Primary Hospice Palliative Care Teams within an agency/facility, Secondary Expert Teams or Tertiary Expert Teams.

1. Case Manager

The role of the Community Case Manager in Palliative Care includes:

Assessment:
- To conduct a thorough assessment, determine eligibility for CCAC services and to work with the person and family to determine the person's needs, and goals of care

- Assessment takes place in the person's home, hospital or in an appropriate setting.

Information and linking:
- To provide information about services that are provided by the CCAC as funded by the Ministry of Health and Long Term Care

- To provide information regarding other appropriate community resources i.e. hospice and to link the person and family with these resources as appropriate.

- To act as a resource and advocate to assist the person and family to navigate through the health care system.

Service Planning:
- To work with the person and family to determine what services are required to meet the person's and family's goals of care in each domain as outlined by the *A Model to Guide Hospice Palliative Care* (Ferris et al., 2002).

Implementation of the Service Plan:

- To set up a service plan based on the person's needs and refer to contracted service providers as outlined by the Ministry of Health / Long Term Care Act Regulations. Services that may be provided include: nursing, physiotherapy, occupational therapy, speech language pathology, dietician, social work, and personal support worker

- To ensure that appropriate supplies and medical equipment are made available.

Reassessment and Evaluation:

- To collaborate with the client's interdisciplinary individualized care team to monitor and reassess needs ongoing

- To ensure that the service plan remains up-to-date and revise the plan as needed when the person's condition and goals of care change. This may mean adding or discontinuing services and increasing or decreasing the amount of services

- To ensure that the care team is aware of the person's death

- To ensure that equipment is removed from the home

- To provide information and referral for bereavement support as appropriate.

2. Clergy / Spiritual Pastoral Care

Role of the Clergy and Pastoral Care:

- To assess the spiritual needs of the person

- To support the person as he or she searches to find meaning and hope in changing circumstances

- To provide opportunity for the person to experience meaningful rituals, sacramental ministry, and prayer

- To participate with the team in ethical decision-making

- To provide grief and bereavement support for person/family/caregiver team.

3. Hospice/Palliative Care Volunteers

Role of the Volunteer:

- To provide practical assistance in meeting the complex needs of the person

- To provide support across various settings

- To listen to the cares and concerns of the person

- To share information disclosed with appropriate service providers and/or volunteer co-ordinator

- To provide information to the person regarding services available

- To advocate for access to services that will meet the person's expressed wishes.

4. Nurse

Role of the Nurse:
- To function within the scope of practice of the College of Nurses of Ontario

- To perform a holistic assessment of the person and support network to identify issues in each of the domains of issues as outlined in the Model to Guide Hospice Palliative Care

- To engage in therapeutic encounters that include assessment, information sharing, decision-making, care planning, care delivery, and confirmation related to each identified issue

- To collaborate with other team members to provide the most appropriate services and maximum quality of life for the person and family.

- To perform delegated medical therapies such as parenteral medication, wound dressing and the maintenance of catheters, and percutaneous tubes

- To collaborate with the physician to monitor and manage disease symptoms and the effects of medical therapy

- To foster the autonomy of the person

- To empower and advocate for the person

- To promote efficient utilization of resources

- To promote opportunities for debriefing and resolution of grief among professional and volunteer caregivers.

Role of the Palliative Pain and Symptom Management Consultant Secondary or Tertiary Clinical Consultant (Ferris et al., 2002):
- To provide a telephone or onsite consultation service for team members related to palliative care and pain and symptom management

- To provide education, training and mentorship for primary clinicians

- To provide up to date, research based and best practice information and guidelines related to palliative care and pain and symptom management on request

- To assist communities to develop hospice palliative care services that will meet local needs

- To promote networking of existing palliative care resources throughout the district

- To advocate for the person in need of pain and symptom management.

Secondary Expert:
- Is expert in hospice palliative care

- Is an experienced member of a designated hospice palliative care team/unit or program

- Supports primary providers in every setting where persons and families receive care.

Tertiary Expert:
- Is an expert practitioner and researcher in hospice palliative care.

Role of the tertiary expert in addition to the above mentioned:
- To consult with secondary experts and primary providers on difficult to manage cases

- To educate secondary and tertiary experts

- To conduct research

- To develop advocacy strategies.

5. Occupational Therapist

Role of the Occupational Therapist:
- To determine the person's desired goals related to daily activity in self care, productivity and leisure
- To assist the person to maintain quality of life through enabling him or her to achieve personal objectives/goals
- To assess loss of mobility; ambulation, bed mobility, transfers, assistive devices, home safety, fall risks, and range of motion
- To recommend and teach the use of assistive devices and specialized equipment to facilitate optimum physical function and comfort
- To ensure that the person is safe within his or her environment
- To anticipate the person's changing status and make appropriate recommendations to minimize changes to care routine
- To advise the person regarding energy conservation techniques to maximize limited energy resources to meaningful activity
- To provide appropriate recommendations for pain and pressure relief or reduction through positioning, lift up and transfer techniques and relaxation exercises
- To increase the ease of handling of the person by supporting caregivers and promoting safety for the person.

6. Personal Support Worker and Health Care Aide

Role of the Personal Support Worker/Health Care Aide:
- To assist with activities of daily living as required: personal care, nutrition, light housekeeping, laundry, respite
- To observe and report to professional service providers and/or supervisors any changes in physical symptoms and emotional responses of the person
- To participate, as a valued member of the health care team, in development and implementation of the care plan
- To assist and support caregivers in the provision of care to the person
- To provide holistic support and advocate as necessary to ensure that the person's needs are met
- To communicate effectively with team members
- To document observations.

7. Pharmacist

Role of the Pharmacist:
- To prepare, dispense and distribute medications to meet the person's specific needs
- To complete a medication assessment, by reviewing the medication profile in order to identify actual or potential drug related problems
- To collaborate with the person, family, and other service providers to ensure that the person's medication needs are met
- To provide education about medications to the person, family and caregivers in order to optimize medication use and adherence and to minimize potential risks of toxicity.
- To develop and implement a pharmacy care plan based on symptom management and drug related needs, with follow-up and outcome monitoring
- To advocate on behalf of the person for optimal medication use
- To act as an easily accessible resource for medication and therapy-related questions.

8. Family Physician

Several physicians may be involved in the care of the person throughout the illness trajectory. It is important to the person's well-being that the family physician be aware of the condition, needs and expectations of the person as the disease progresses. The family physician is the most appropriate person to coordinate the medical care during the end-of-life stage of a life threatening illness (A Colloquium on the Care of the Dying Patient, 1996).

One of the most fundamental and urgent needs of the dying person is to have a physician who will not only assume responsibility for medical care but is also prepared to offer a listening ear and to serve as a skilled and sensitive professional in a situation of great sadness for all involved (A Colloquium on the Care of the Dying Patient, 1996).

Role of the Family Physician:
Adapted from College of Physicians and Surgeons of Ontario, Decision Making for the End-of-life: Role of the Physician (2006).

- To assess the medical care needs of the person and family
- To provide care that fulfills the person's/family's goals
- To be compassionate and respectful
- To help the person/family cope with physical, psychological, social and spiritual needs and relieve unnecessary suffering
- To advocate for meaningful and/or realistic goals of care involving early discussion of diagnosis and prognosis and the potential benefits, burdens, and risks associated with various therapies and with the refusal of therapy
- To provide ongoing medical care, support and guidance
- To understand the impact of culture and religion on the person's personal choices
- To ask about and seek to incorporate the person's and family's choices, values, beliefs and goals in decisions for end-of-life
- To be aware of community palliative care resources
- To actively participate in case conferences
- To encourage the discussion of the importance of advance care planning and, as the illness progresses, reassess with the person and family on an ongoing basis
- To ensure that other members of the care team are informed about treatment decisions relating to resuscitation and life support and that discussions are carefully documented in the health record
- To collaborate with other members of the team in devising a plan of care
- To communicate in a timely manner with the person and family concerning treatment options, assessment of options made by the health care team, supportive services and palliative care resources
- To facilitate access to interdisciplinary pain and symptom management, palliative and supportive care
- To allow the person to experience as dignified a death as possible
- To endeavour to honour the last wishes of the person wherever it is possible to do so
- To designate a substitute physician whenever he or she is not available, ensuring that such designate is appraised of the situation
- To attend to the certification of the death, facilitate the removal of the body, and provide emotional support to the bereaved within a reasonable time after death has ensued. The procedure and time frame will have been discussed with the service providers and caregivers prior to the death.
- To plan for bereavement follow-up care as appropriate to family needs.

Role of the Palliative Care Physician Consultant:
- To act as the medical advisor/consultant on the agency/facility/community Palliative Care Team

- To act as a liaison between the medical staff and the Palliative Care Team

- To act, whenever necessary, as an advocate for the person and family referred to the Palliative Care Team

- To participate in team meetings/case conferences as required

- To promote and participate in palliative care education of all services providers/caregivers

- To encourage the emotional, psychosocial, and spiritual well being of staff, volunteers and others working in palliative care.

9. Physician Assistant

The Personal Assistant (PA) role is currently being introduced to the Ontario health care system. Physician assistants (PAs) are skilled health professionals who support physicians in a range of health care settings. They work alongside physicians, nurses, nurse practitioners and other members of the interprofessional health care team. The specific duties of the PA vary depending on the individual competencies of the PA, the supervising physician's area of practice, and the types of duties that the supervising physician chooses to assign. Examples include:

- Conduct patient interviews and take medical histories

- Perform physical examinations

- Perform certain controlled acts delegated to them by a physician

- Initiate and interpret tests, analyze data, implement and evaluate plans of care. Effectively manage the plan of care for each patient based on clinical knowledge, data, patient preference and benefits to the patient

- Provide counselling.

10. Physiotherapist

Role of the Physiotherapist:
- To act as a complementary part of the professional team, and help set and achieve the person's goals

- To assess circulation, chest status, edema, DVT, skin breakdown due to loss of mobility, and pain

- To manage symptoms, reduce pain and provide support with the use of appropriate modalities such as TENS, ultrasound, acupuncture, heat/cold, proper positioning

- To improve mobility by assessing for proper aids, teaching transfers and teaching strengthening exercises

- To deal with respiratory function with the use of vibrators, breathing techniques, mucociliary clearance, and/or oxygen saturation testing with exercise

- To improve skin integrity via the use of support or compression bandaging, use of compression pump and use of wound management techniques

- To teach relaxation techniques.

11. Recreation Therapist

Role of the Recreation Therapist:
- To provide activities/programs/social visits to residents commensurate with and appropriate to their mental and physical status

- To coordinate with care plan team to provide maximum opportunities to enhance quality of life e.g. complementary therapies

- To promote activities that involve the search for meaning, confronting fears, dealing with the loss of control, and other issues of loss.

- To address the dying person's negative feelings; threats to self esteem and to help restore a sense of control, contributing to an improved quality of life.

- To reduce boredom, foster a sense of accomplishment and enhance psycho-social supports within the person's community

- To inform, invite and provide special escort to activities and programs of choice.

- To modify activities/programs/social visits offered to match resident's mental and physical changes.

- To provide guidance to staff as to appropriate recreational activities.

- To provide guidance and support to families as to appropriate recreational activities to match resident's status

- To provide for "final wish" opportunities to residents as tolerated and feasible.

12. Registered Dietician

Role of the Registered Dietician:
- To assess nutritional status, history and goals of the person

- To develop an individual nutritional care plan with the person based on factors affecting adequacy of intake, therapeutic issues and physiological state

- To educate and support the person, caregivers and other service providers

- To monitor the effect of interventions, disease progression, concerns of the person and adapt the care plan as required

- To advise the person of available funding for the use of supplements or equipment

- To assist the person in decisions regarding nutrition support and alternative nutrition strategies.

13. Respiratory Therapist

Role of the Respiratory Therapist:

- To assist in developing a plan to address respiratory insufficiency – thus optimizing comfort through appropriate intervention with oxygen therapy, inhalation therapy, and suction

- To provide counselling in breathing techniques, mucociliary clearance, activity tolerance, and medication – as appropriate

- To advise the person/family/caregivers of available funding – as well as discussing possible alternatives where no funding sources exist i.e. self pay

- To revise the care plan as the disease progresses

- To instruct the person, caregivers and services providers in the operation, maintenance and precautions of appropriate equipment/care plan

- To communicate effectively with team members in case conferences, with timely report, assessment and other related documentation

- To be available on a 24 hour emergency basis to address equipment malfunctions.

14. Social Worker

Role of the Social Worker:
- To assess psychosocial needs and develop a care plan to meet identified needs

- To explore emotional basis for intractable pain and assist person in developing coping strategies for the management of such pain

- To assist team members with interactions with clients

- To assist around practical issues such as finances, will, Power of Attorney and funeral planning

- To provide individual and family counselling as necessary.

15. Speech-Language Pathologist

Role of the Speech-Language Pathologist:
- To assess present and future communication needs and/or swallowing needs of the person

- To education the person, caregivers and service providers on the expectation of future communication abilities and/or swallowing difficulties

- To assist in developing a plan and teaching strategies to meet future communication and/or swallowing needs.

Acknowlegements

Chapter Three

Domain: Disease Management

Disease Management

- Primary diagnosis, prognosis, evidence

- Secondary diagnosis (e.g. dementia, substance use)

- Co-morbidities (e.g. delirium, seizures)

- Adverse events (e.g. side effects)

- Allergies

Person and Family

- Demographics

- Culture

- Personal values, beliefs, practices and strengths

- Developmental stage, education, literacy

- Disabilities

Ferris et al., 2002

Understanding Disease Management

An understanding of the disease process and its treatment will help the caregiver to be effective in facilitating a more positive experience of the illness for both the person and family. Although cancer is a disease commonly associated with hospice palliative care, there are many other diseases that merit a similar approach to care. Diseases such as ALS (amyotrophic lateral sclerosis, or Lou Gehrig's disease), liver disease, heart disease, COPD (chronic obstructive pulmonary disease), renal failure, AIDS (Acquired Immune Deficiency Syndrome), and Alzheimer Disease are also progressive and life-limiting.

Navigating the Journey

The course of most progressive life-limiting diseases is unpredictable. Throughout the illness journey, including at the end stage, palliative care is closely tailored to the actual issues that are identified in each of the domains of issues. In many illnesses, treatments aimed at prolonging life are often aggressively administered up to the point of death. The pediatric palliative care guidelines refer to this as ruthless obstinacy. Discussing the burdens and benefits of treatment interventions all along the illness trajectory and ensuring that individuals are aware that they can choose to withhold or withdraw life-prolonging treatments at any time is part of good palliative care. Defining clear goals of care assists in ensuring that the person's wishes are honoured.

The various choices that a person with a life-limiting illness is called upon to make along the illness trajectory are illustrated in the "road map" below.

NAVIGATING LIFE'S JOURNEY
A Roadmap to Support Decision Making

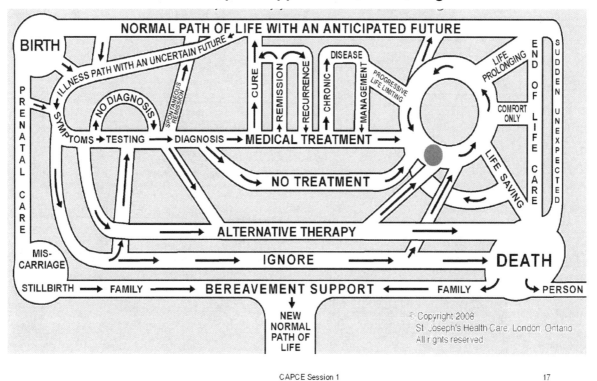

The "road map" represents the various routes and the decision-making points along the way; from the point of onset of symptoms to the ultimate destination which is death for the person with the disease and bereavement for the family. Decisions are made as to whether or not to have various tests, what treatments to accept, whether or not to explore alternative treatments and when to withhold or withdraw treatment. The formal caregiver is present along the illness path to be an advocate, to give information, encouragement, and support as well as good bedside care.

Another way of looking at an illness trajectory is in terms of stages. The Palliative Performance Scale (PPS) is an 11-point scale designed to measure patients' performance status in 10% decrements from 100% (healthy) to 0% (death) based on five observable parameters: ambulation, ability to do activities, self-care, food/fluid intake, and consciousness level. www.victoriahospice.org/care_medical.html

Stages based on PPS scores.

1. Stable Stage when the PPS scores range from 100% - 70%

2. Transitional Stage when the PPS scores range from 60% - 40%

3. End-of-Life Stage when the PPS scores range from 30%-0%

The PPS is a reliable and valid tool researched in the cancer population that can help caregivers identify and track care needs as they change with disease progression. The PPS provides a framework for measuring progressive decline over the course of the illness; it also provides a "best guess" projection of length of survival (i.e. suggests if a person is moving closer to death) and serves as a communication tool for the team. The PPS can also serve as a workload measurement tool as a person who scores between 0-40% usually requires increased hands-on care and family members need more support compared to those persons with higher PPS scores.

The table used to determine the PPS score is illustrated below. Instructions on use of the PPS follow on the next page.

Palliative Performance Scale (PPSv2) Version 2

PPS Level	Ambulation	Activity & Evidence of Disease	Self-Care	Intake	Conscious Level
100%	Full	Normal activity & work No evidence of disease	Full	Normal	Full
90%	Full	Normal activity & work Some evidence of disease	Full	Normal	Full
80%	Full	Normal activity with effort Some evidence of disease	Full	Normal or reduced	Full
70%	Reduced	Unable normal job/work Significant disease	Full	Normal or reduced	Full
60%	Reduced	Unable hobby/house work Significant disease	Occasional assistance necessary	Normal or reduced	Full or Confusion
50%	Mainly Sit/Lie	Unable to do any work Extensive disease	Considerable assistance required	Normal or reduced	Full or Confusion
40%	Mainly in Bed	Unable to do most activity Extensive disease	Mainly assistance	Normal or reduced	Full or Drowsy +/- Confusion
30%	Totally Bed Bound	Unable to do any activity Extensive disease	Total Care	Normal or reduced	Full or Drowsy +/- Confusion
20%	Totally Bed Bound	Unable to do any activity Extensive disease	Total Care	Minimal to Sips	Full or Drowsy +/- Confusion
10%	Totally Bed Bound	Unable to do any activity Extensive disease	Total Care	Mouth care Only	Drowsy or Coma +/- Confusion
0%	Death	-	-	-	-

Instructions for Use of PPS (see also definition of terms)

1. PPS scores are determined by reading horizontally at each level to find a 'best fit' for the individual that is then assigned as the PPS% score.

2. Begin at the left column and read downwards until the appropriate ambulation level is reached, then read across to the next column and downwards again until the activity/evidence of disease is located. These steps are repeated until all five columns are covered before assigning the actual PPS for that individual. In this way, 'leftward' columns (columns to the left of any specific column) are 'stronger' determinants and generally take precedence over others.

   Example 1: The person who spends the majority of the day sitting or lying down due to fatigue from advanced disease and requires considerable assistance to walk even for short distances but who is otherwise fully conscious with good intake would be scored at PPS 50%.

   Example 2: An individual who has become paralyzed and quadriplegic requiring total care would be PPS 30%. Although this person may be placed in a wheelchair (and perhaps seem initially to be at 50%), the score is 30% because he or she would be otherwise totally bed bound due to the disease or complication if it were not for caregivers providing total care including lift/transfer. The person may have normal intake and full conscious level.

   Example 3: However, if the person in example 2 was paraplegic and bed bound but still able to do some self-care such as feed self, then the PPS would be higher at 40% or 50% since he or she is not 'total care'.

3. PPS scores are in 10% increments only. Sometimes, there are several columns easily placed at one level but one or two which seem better at a higher or lower level. One then needs to make a 'best fit' decision. Choosing a 'half-fit' value of PPS 45%, for example, is not correct. The combination of clinical judgment and 'leftward precedence' is used to determine whether 40% or 50% is the more accurate score for that person.

Definition of Terms for PPS
(Victoria Hospice Society, 2001)

Some of the terms have similar meanings with the differences being more readily apparent as one reads horizontally across each row to find an overall 'best fit' using all five columns.

1. Ambulation

The items **'mainly sit/lie,' 'mainly in bed,'** and **'totally bed bound'** are clearly similar. The subtle differences are related to items in the self-care column. For example, 'totally bed bound' at PPS 30% is due to either profound weakness or paralysis such that the person not only can't get out of bed but is also unable to do any self-care. The difference between 'sit, lie, and bed' is proportionate to the amount of time the person is able to sit up versus need to lie down.

'Reduced ambulation' is located at the PPS 70% and PPS 60% level. By using the adjacent column, the reduction of ambulation is tied to inability to carry out their normal job, work occupation or some hobbies or housework activities. The person is still able to walk and transfer independently but at PPS 60% needs occasional assistance.

2. Activity & Extent of Disease

'Some', 'significant', and **'extensive'** disease refer to physical and investigative evidence which shows degrees of progression. For example in breast cancer, a local recurrence would imply 'some' disease, one or two metastases in the lung or bone would imply 'significant' disease, whereas multiple metastases in lung, bone, liver, brain, hypercalcemia or other major complications would be 'extensive' disease. The extent may also refer to progression of disease despite active treatments. Using PPS in AIDS, 'some' may mean the shift from HIV to AIDS, 'significant' implies progression in physical decline, new or difficult symptoms and laboratory findings with low counts. 'Extensive' refers to one or more serious complications with or without continuation of active antiretrovirals, antibiotics, etc.

The above extent of disease is also judged in context with the ability to maintain one's work and hobbies or activities. Decline in activity may mean the person still plays golf but adjusts from playing 18 holes to 9 holes, or just a par 3, or to backyard putting. People who enjoy walking will gradually reduce the distance covered, although they may continue trying, sometimes even close to death (e.g. trying to walk the halls).

3. Self-Care

'Occasional assistance' means that most of the time the person is able to transfer out of bed, walk, wash, toilet and eat by his or her own means, but that on occasion (perhaps once daily or a few times weekly) minor assistance is required.

'Considerable assistance' means that regularly every day the individual needs help, usually by one person, to do some of the activities noted above. For example, the person needs help to get to the bathroom but is then able to brush his or her teeth or wash at least hands and face. Food will often need to be cut into edible sizes but the person is then able to eat of his or her own accord.

'Mainly assistance' is a further extension of 'considerable'. Using the above example, the person now needs help getting up but also needs assistance with washing, but can usually eat with minimal or no help. This may fluctuate according to fatigue during the day.

'Total care' means that the person is completely unable to eat without help, toilet or do any self-care. Depending on the clinical situation, the person may or may not be able to chew and swallow food once prepared and fed to him or her.

4. Intake

Changes in intake are quite obvious with **'normal intake'** referring to the person's usual eating habits while healthy. **'Reduced'** means any reduction from that and is highly variable according to the unique individual circumstances. **'Minimal'** refers to very small amounts, usually pureed or liquid, which are well below nutritional sustenance.

5. Conscious Level

'Full consciousness' implies full alertness and orientation with good cognitive abilities in various domains of thinking, memory, etc. **'Confusion'** is used to denote presence of either delirium or dementia and is a reduced level of consciousness. It may be mild, moderate or severe with multiple possible etiologies. **'Drowsiness'** implies fatigue, drug side effects, delirium or closeness to death and is sometimes included in the term stupor. **'Coma'** in this context is the absence of response to verbal or physical stimuli; some reflexes may or may not remain. The depth of coma may fluctuate throughout a 24 hour period.

Scoring of PPS scores should be initiated when there are no further interventions whose goal is cure or remission available to the person with a life-threatening illness.

1. In the home setting
   • Good practice is to complete the PPS at each visit

2. In the hospital or palliative care unit setting
   • Good practice is to complete the PPS at the same time each day

3. In a long-term care home setting
   • Good practice is to complete the PPS on admission, quarterly, and daily when a score of 30% is not maintained concurrently for 72 hours and daily for scores of 20% and lower.

Who Should Complete the PPS?

- The PPS can be completed by any regulated health care provider. It is anticipated, that in most cases, the PPS will be completed by a registered nurse or a registered practical nurse. All team members are responsible for observing the person carefully and identifying and reporting any changes in ambulation, activity and evidence of disease, self-care, intake and consciousness that would indicate a change in the PPS score.

Where to Document the PPS

- The PPS score is transcribed into the health care record, on the flow sheet or in the progress notes as per organizational policy.

The Palliative Performance System was researched in the cancer population but has application in other illnesses in terms of measuring functional status and as a workload measurement.

An understanding of the specific disease process and commonly experienced symptoms will promote early identification of issues. Only when issues are identified can proper interventions be initiated and evaluated. Being mindful of what stage of the illness trajectory the person is in and being sensitive to the lived experience of the person and family will promote appropriate disease and symptom management throughout the illness trajectory. Identification of the final or terminal phase of the illness creates an opportunity for formal caregivers to prepare the person and family for the inevitable death.

Palliative Illnesses

The following chart includes information related to common progressive life-limiting illnesses along with suggested disease management interventions and some of the common symptoms experienced. The symptoms may occur prior to diagnosis as well as throughout the illness trajectory.

Acquired Immune Deficiency Syndrome (AIDS)

The human immunodeficiency virus is a retrovirus that causes acquired immune deficiency syndrome. Before the advent of antiretroviral treatment, AIDS resulted in death within a few years. Now with treatment, it is a chronic progressive illness that is still incurable. Symptom recognition and control are important for quality of life and palliative care should accompany disease management throughout the trajectory. Regardless of how the disease was acquired, as life expectancy is extended, infected individuals are developing more malignancies and organ failure related to the toxicity of the antiretroviral treatment itself. It is important that the person's goals of care be reviewed throughout the illness to ensure that treatment to prolong life is in keeping with the person's goals. End stage events with this disease can happen quickly. It is not unusual for the person with HIV/AIDS to be admitted, intubated, and dead within hours or days. (Alexandra in Emmanuel and Librach 2007)

Trajectory	Interventions	Commonly Experienced Symptoms
Gradual decline over months or years. • Stages • Early • Progressive • Advanced • Terminal	• Medications to manage disease • Antibiotics for opportunistic infections • Chemo and Radiation for related cancers • Supportive Care	• Fatigue, fever, pain (especially in hands and feet), nausea, diarrhea, sadness/depression, sleep problems, skin problems, cough, headaches, anorexia, weight loss, dyspnea • Side effects of antiretrovirals include loss of facial fat, muscle wasting, anorexia, myalgias, nausea and eventually unresponsiveness and sepsis

---

Alzheimer Disease

Alzheimer is the most common form of dementia. It is a chronic, progressive and incurable neurodegenerative disease that results in much loss and significant suffering for both the person and family. As in other forms of dementia, impairments in memory, judgment, language, behaviours and function occur over time. Prevalence increases with age and the population of persons with dementia is expected to increase 10 fold over the next 40 years. Failure to recognize neurodegenerative illnesses as progressive and incurable may result in inadequate symptom management and end-of-life care. Prognosis guidelines focus on functional indicators such as the Functional Assessment Staging Scale. A combination of functional and nutritional impairment is associated with shorter survival times. Acute illnesses and hospitalizations are associated with poorer prognosis. A study of demented patients with a diagnosis of hip fracture or pneumonia found that half the patients died within 6 months. (Modi, Kapo, Casarett in Emmanuel and Librach 2007)

Trajectory	Interventions	Commonly Experienced Symptoms
Usually a slow steady decline. Advance care planning is helpful in setting goals and planning for disease progression	• Medications to slow progression (efficacy in late stages is questionable) • Symptom management and supportive care	• Early: confusion, forgetfulness, depression, anxiety, insomnia • Later: visual and aural hallucinations, paranoia, agitation and restlessness are seen in up to 80% of cases. • Other behaviours that may be exhibited are physical and verbal aggression and sexually inappropriate actions. • Impairment in abilities related to ADLs and IADLs, pacing and wandering are all progressive over time. • **RULE OUT DELIRIUM** whenever there is an acute change in behaviour

Heart Disease: Congestive Heart Failure(CHF)

Heart failure is increasingly viewed as a chronic disease that can be managed. It is a fluctuating life-limiting illness and there may not be a discrete point at which it is deemed terminal. Both physicians and persons with heart disease are not inclined to consider the possibility of treatment failure. With each exacerbation, prognosis is unpredictable. The terminal phase is not clearly defined and sudden death is frequent. Because of the high symptom burden, palliative care has much to offer to this group of persons. Pneumonia is common in persons who are debilitated by heart failure and treatment depends on the person's goals of care. Frank conversations about likely symptoms and prognosis need to be carried out at multiple points along the trajectory. If the person has an Automated Implantable Cardiac Defibrillator (AICD), a discussion about deactivation needs to happen when dying is evident. Studies have shown a low percentage of person's with CHF having a DNR as opposed to illnesses such as cancer and dementia which is probably indicative of a lack of discussion about goals of care and prognosis. (Hauser and Bonow in Emmanuel and Librach 2007)

Trajectory	Interventions	Commonly Experienced Symptoms
Multiple stages during which a combination of disease managing therapies and symptom directed therapies are appropriate	• ACE inhibitors • Beta Blockers • Diuretics • Digoxin The above medications have symptomatic benefits and so should be maintained • There is no evidence to support oxygen as a life prolonging treatment • Opioids or sedatives for symptoms • Supportive care	• Dyspnea related to angina • Dyspnea may be due to a comorbid condition such as COPD, asthma, • Fatigue may be exacerbated by sleep apnea • Pain other than angina is generally related to other conditions such as arthritis • Depression

---

Amyotrophic Lateral Sclerosis (ALS)

ALS is one form of neurodegenerative disease; others include Multiple Sclerosis, Parkinson Disease, Muscular Dystrophy. ALS can manifest in different ways depending on the groupings of neurons involved. Motor neurons in the upper spine control the arms and hands while neurons in the lower spine control the legs and feet. Motor neurons in the brainstem control speech chewing and swallowing. Symptoms are vague at first and the person and family need support all throughout the trajectory from the time of testing to the end of life. Symptom management is critical to enhance quality of life. The health care providers need to be alert to subtle changes and attempt to be one step ahead in order to avoid crises from arising. (Jones and Colman in Emmanuel and Librach 2007)

Trajectory	Interventions	Commonly Experienced Symptoms
Average survival from diagnosis is 3 years	• With permission refer to ALS Society • Arrange home care services early • Frequent assessments • Medications to manage the symptoms • Supportive care	• Symptoms that result from muscle weakness include: muscle cramps, spasticity, dysarthria (difficulty with speech), dysphagia (difficulty swallowing), drooling, dyspnea, pain, choking, anxiety, depression • Indirect symptoms include pain, constipation, nausea, sleep disturbance and depression • Some persons with ALS may develop frontotemperal dementia that results in changes in personality, social withdrawal, finding words, difficulty as well as problems with organization • A syndrome of pathological laughter or tears can occur

---

Renal Disease

Persons with renal failure who are on dialysis have a significantly shortened life expectancy, high symptom burden (on average 9 symptoms) and multiple co morbid conditions. Diabetes, cardiac disease, and anemia often are forerunners of renal failure. Almost all individuals with end stage renal disease who stop renal dialysis die within a month, yet very few are referred for palliative care. There is a growing trend to have nephrologists and their staff acquire education and skill in palliative care so that symptoms can be better addressed and advance care planning with goal setting can be part of the treatment discussions for those with renal disease. The age at which dialysis is begun has become older and older persons on dialysis withdraw treatment more often than younger persons. (Moss in Emmanuel and Librach 2007)

Trajectory	Interventions	Commonly Experienced Symptoms
5 year survival rate on dialysis is 33%. When dialysis is withdrawn death from uremia usually occurs within 8 to 12 days although persons have lived for up to a month. Death is usually gentle with increasing somnolence as death approaches	• Dialysis • Peritoneal dialysis • Hemodialysis • Kidney transplant • Symptom management and supportive care	• Early: muscular pains, edema, weakness and fatigue • Later, following initiation of dialysis: chest pain, bone or joint pain, difficulty becoming sexually aroused, trouble falling asleep, muscle cramps, itching, fatigue

Chronic Obstructive Pulmonary Disease (COPD)

COPD is one of many progressive respiratory illnesses. Others include pulmonary fibrosis, Cystic Fibrosis, Occupational Lung Diseases etc. COPD is the 4th leading cause of death in the world. It is a progressive life-limiting illness. Primary disease management includes combinations of short and long acting bronchodilators, corticosteroids, oxygen, pulmonary rehabilitation and preventative measures such as vaccinations for flu and pneumonia. Treatments are aimed at improving pulmonary function tests, exercise capacity, function and symptoms. The summary of studies from the Association of Palliative Medicine Science Committee regarding persons with COPD advises that there is equivocal evidence for the use of long term oxygen at rest for palliation of dyspnea. Oxygen may be of benefit for decreasing breathlessness associated with exercise. The effect of oxygen on quality of life during ambulation cannot be predicted by patient characteristics. It must be based on a trial. Opiates and benzodiazepines are very helpful in the management of dyspnea and the accompanying anxiety. Analysis of numerous trials involving nebulized opioids suggests that it has no role in the relief of dyspnea. (Groninger and Muir in Emmanuel and Librach 2007)

Trajectory	Interventions	Commonly Experienced Symptoms
COPD involves inevitable decline and increasingly frequent hospital admissions to treat exacerbations, often with extensive periods of ventilator support	• Prevention of infection • Chest physiotherapy • Medications to manage symptoms • Surgery: lung transplant • Ventilators • Supportive care	• dyspnea • Anxiety • Depression • Fatigue • Confusion • Cough

Liver Disease: Cirrhosis and Fibrosis

Cirrhosis is a progressive liver disease, and damage sustained to the liver is irreversible. In chronic liver disease, there is gradual destruction of liver tissue over time. However, with proper nutrition, avoidance of certain toxins (i.e., alcohol), vitamin supplementation, and management of cirrhosis complications, further liver damage can often be delayed or stopped. In severe cases of cirrhosis, liver transplantation may be considered. Cirrhosis is the 7th leading cause of death in the U.S. Because of chronic liver damage, functioning tissue is replaced by scar tissue and blood flow through the liver is diminished. Nutrients, hormones, drugs and poisons are then not effectively processed and other functions are inhibited. The most common cause of cirrhosis is alcohol abuse. A few of the other causes include hepatitis and other viruses, use of certain drugs, chemical exposure, bile duct obstruction, autoimmune diseases. Fibrosis is the growth of scar tissue due to infection, inflammation, injury, or even healing. Fibrosis in the liver can inhibit the organ's proper functioning and usually results in cirrhosis. (University of Maryland Medical Centre 2008)

Trajectory	Interventions	Symptoms
Usually slow and tedious process	• Management of: • Electrolytes • Bleeds • Infections • Ascites (abdominal fluid) • Encephalopathy • Supportive care • Liver transplant	• Depend on severity of disease • Abnormal nerve function • Ascites, itching • Coughing up or vomiting blood • Jaundice • Kidney failure • Muscle loss, weakness • Liver encephalopathy (confusion) • Fatigue, lack of stamina, • Decreased appetite • Abdominal bloating

Cancer

Cancer is a genetic disease in which the regulation, characteristics and function of normal cells is abnormal. Genetic mutations allow malignant cells to gain advantage over normal cells and grow uncontrollably. The development of cancer involves many steps that take place over many years. Although some cancers are inherited, most are due to a series of somatic mutations. Environmental and personal factors can affect the development of cancer. Environmental factors include chemicals, smoking, excessive alcohol intake, radiation (ionizing e.g. x-rays and ultraviolet e.g. sun), chronic irritation, viral agents and dietary influences. Personal factors include immune system function, advancing age, failure of the body's surveillance system that detects the presence of foreign invaders and destroys them. Some individuals have a genetic predisposition that influences the carcinogenetic process. Race is a genetically determined characteristic that plays a role in cancer incidence.

Cancer incidence and survival can be related to socioeconomic factors as well.

(Klem and Hurst 2009)

Many types of cancer cells have the ability to spread or metastasize. Some parts of the body are more apt to develop metastases than others. It is quite common for cancer to spread in the liver, lungs, and bones, but rare for cancer to spread in skin. Each type of cancer has its own pattern for spread. Cancer can spread via the blood stream, the lymphatic system or by local invasion. Metastasis can happen accidentally when a biopsy is done or during surgery when a malignant cell may actually drip from a needle or instrument. This spread is rare and is caused by implantation or inoculation

Cancers that metastasize remain the same cancer i.e. cancer of the breast that spreads to the lung remains cancer of the breast; it is not lung cancer.

Breast Cancer can include: the nipple, areola, ducts, lobules, adipose tissue, pectoralis minor and major muscles and associated lymph nodes. It is the most common cancer in women in industrialized countries and the incidence increases with age. (Payne 2009)

Metastasizes to	Treatments	Commonly Experienced Symptoms
Bone Lung Liver Brain Trajectory: depends on staging at the time of diagnosis	• Surgery • Radiation • Chemotherapy • Hormone therapy	• Depend on locations of cancer metasteses • Lymphedema • Pain • Fatigue • Shortness of breath • Loss of appetite • Headaches

---

Central Nervous System Malignancies are cancers of the brain or spinal cord. Primary brain tumours originate from neuronal or non neuronal tissue in the brain or spinal cord.

Many tumours of the CNS are metastatic arising from primary tumours of the lung, breast, colon, skin (melanomas) and kidney. (Page and Federoff 2007)

Trajectory	Interventions	Commonly Experienced Symptoms
Variable, depends on tumour type	Based on tumour type but includes: • Surgery • Radiation • Chemotherapy • Steroids • Anticonvulsants	• Increased intercraial pressure leading to headache, nausea, vomiting, altered level of consciousness and seizures • Depending on tumour location there may be weakness, sensory changes, personality changes and endocrine abnormalities

Gastrointestinal malignancies include anal cancer, biliary cancer, gallbladder cancer, colon and rectal cancer, esophageal cancer, gastric cancer, liver cancer, pancreatic cancer.

(Grande, Hoyer, Keith, Agbajana, Smith-Zamiska, Roll 2009)

Trajectory	Interventions	Commonly Experienced Symptoms
Variable, depends on tumour location and staging at diagnosis. Pancreatic cancer generally has a poor prognosis, while anal cancer, if caught early, is curable	• Surgery • Radiation • Chemotherapy	Depends on site: • Weight loss • Anorexia • Nausea • Vomiting • Pain • Dysphagia • Jaundice • Itching

Genitourinary Cancers include cancers of the bladder, penis, prostate, kidney, and testicles. (Collins, Bunch 2009)

Metastatic sites	Interventions	Commonly Experienced Symptoms
Bladder • Lymphatic system, lung, bone, liver, brain	• **Surgery** • **Radiation** • **Chemotherapy**	**Bladder** • Frequency • Urgency • Dysuria • Altered stream • Bone pain, flank and pelvic . **Penile** • Small papules to fungating lesions.
Prostate • bone, lungs, brain		**Prostate** • Frequency, hesitancy, decreased stream, nocturia • Bone pain, usually ribs, back and hips related to bone mets .
Kidney-metastasizes to bone, liver, lung, brain and distant lymph nodes.		**Kidney** • Flank pain • Hematuria • Weight loss • Fatigue • Anemia.
Testicular Via lymphatic system to retroperitoneal lymph nodes. Distant sites include lung, liver, skeleton, brain		**Testicular** • Swelling, nodules, pain, hardness, feeling of heaviness • Advanced – back or abdominal pain, weight loss, gynecomastia, supraclavicualar lymphadenopathy, superior vena cava syndrome, urinary obstruction, dyspnea, hemoptysis, bone pain, headaches, seizures

Gynecological Cancers includes cancer of the cervix, endometrial tissue, ovaries, vagina, and vulva. (Bunch 2009)

Metastatic Spread	Interventions	Commonly Experienced Symptoms
Cervical To vaginal mucosa, myometrium, peracervical lymphatics, to common lymph nodes.	• Surgery • Chemotherapy • Radiation • Hormonal Therapy	**Cervical** (is a sexually transmitted disease associated with chronic infection by oncogenic types of HPV) Early symptoms • Vaginal discharge • Painless postcoital spotting Late symptoms • Dysuria, hematuria, rectal bleeding, pain in flank or legs, persistent lower extremity edema, massive hemorrhage, uremia **Endometrial:** • Abnormal vaginal discharge • Postmenopausal bleeding • Pelvic pressure
Ovarian cancer can spread to other abdominal organs.		**Ovarian:** • Vague abdominal discomfort • Dyspepsia • Mild digestive disturbances
Most **vaginal** neoplasms are metastases from other primary sites such as the cervix, vulva and endometrium.		**Vaginal:** • Bloody vaginal discharge • Postcoital spotting • Irregular or post menopausal bleeding • Dysuria • Pelvic pain is a late symptom
Vulvar Local spread		**Vulvar:** • Pruritis • Local pain • Bleeding • Drainage

Head and Neck Cancers include cancer of the larynx, oral cavity, pharynx, salivary glands, thyroid and parathyroid. (Strobl 2009)

Metastatic spread	Interventions	Commonly Experienced Symptoms
Laryngeal: Spreads to regional lymph nodes and bone. Distant metasteses are common.	• Surgery • Radiation • Chemotherapy	**Laryngeal:** • Sore throat, painful swallowing, referred ear pain, weight loss, change in voice quality, hoarseness, difficulty swallowing, dyspnea, stridor throat irritation, hemoptysis
Oral Cavity: Distant metastases possible		**Oral cavity:** • Leukoplakia, ulcers, lump of thickening, feeling of fullness in the throat, dysphagia, jaw swelling, unilateral otalgia (ear pain) without hearing loss, pain, bleeding **Pharangeal:** • Neck mass, nasal obstruction, change in voice quality, sore throat, difficulty swallowing, sense of foreign body in the throat, ear pain, dysphagia, weight loss **Salivary Glands:** • Painless swelling, numbness or weakness in the face, persistent facial pain
Thyroid Cancer Hematogenous and lymphatic spread and distant metasteses are possible	• Surgery • Radioactive Iodine • Radiation • Chemotherapy	**Thyroid and parathyroid tumors:** • Fatigue, weight loss, forgetfulness, renal stones

Leukemias are malignant neoplasms characterized by abnormal proliferation and development of leukocytes which infiltrate bone marrow, peripheral blood and other organs resulting in altered normal cell differentiation. Leukemias (lymphocytic or myelogenous) can be acute or chronic. (Simpson 2009)

	Interventions	Commonly Experienced Symptoms
	• Chemotherapy • Interferon therapy • Radiation therapy • Stem cell transplantation • Surgery to remove enlarged spleen • Bone marrow transplant	• Presenting symptoms are related to bone marrow failure with resulting anaemia, neutropenia, thrombocytopenia or organ fitration with leukemic cells in the spleen, liver and gums. • Malaise • Fatigue • Bone pain especially sternum • Sweats • Bleeding bruising • Pallor, petechiae, eccymosis, lymphadenopathy, spleenomegaly, hepatmegaly, mediastinal mass, abdominal adenopathy

Multiple Myeloma is a cancer of the plasma cell. (Simpson 2009)		
	Interventions	Commonly Experienced Symptoms
Multiple myeloma is seldom curable.	• Bisphosphonates • Supportive care • Pain management • Radiation therapy • Surgery for problematic lytic bone lesions • Chemotherapy • Stem cell transplantation	• No symptoms in the early stages • Pain as a result of osteoporosis and fractures of the lower back and ribs. Other osteoporotic sites are pelvis and skull. • Fatigue from anemia • Recurrent infections particularly pneumonia • Hypercalcemia • Renal damage and potential kidney failure

Lung Cancer is the development of cancer in any area of the lungs or bronchus. It has two main types: small cell lung cancer (SCLC) and non-small cell lung cancer(NSCLC). Tobacco is the primary risk factor. Tiedemann in Newton et al (2009)		
Metastases	Interventions	Commonly Experienced Symptoms
NSCLC • Adenocarcinoma • Squamous carcinoma • Large cell carcinoma Spreads locally and can occlude the bronchial lumens, grow into the pleura and chest wall. It also spreads via the lymphatic system and the blood stream. It finally spreads to bone, liver, adrenal glands and the brain.	• If localized, surgery is the treatment of choice • Radiation therapy • Chemotherapy	• Persistent cough • Shortness of breath • Blood tinged sputum • Chest pain • Hoarseness • Recurrent bronchitis or pneumonia • Pain from bone mets • Fatigue • Anorexia and weight loss • CNS changes • Hypercalcemia
SCLC Few are cured	• Surgery – rare • Radiation • Chemotherapy • Prophylactic brain radiation is controversial • Palliative radiation is done for symptom management	• Same as above

Sarcomas are primary cancers of many different types. Sarcomas arise from tissue called mesemchymal tissue which is the precursor to fibrous tissue, muscle, bone and fat.

Chondrosarcome and Ewing's sarcoma are primary bone cancers and are often curable with treatment.

Kaposi's Sarcoma is a cancer of the lymphatic endothelium and forms vascular channels that fill with blood cells giving it a bruise-like appearance. It is generally not considered to be a true sarcoma which is a tumour arising from connective tissue.

Osteosarcoma is another primary bone cancer. It can be cured but can metastasize to the lung.

Soft tissue sarcomas occur in the supporting tissues and soft tissues of the body e.g. muscle, fat, blood vessels, lymph vessels, nerves and ligaments, tissues around joints, fibrous tissues. There are 50 or more subtypes of soft tissue sarcomas. (Leaby 2009)

Metastases	Interventions	Commonly Experienced Symptoms
Sarcomas can spread throughout the body, although certain sarcomas have more or less of a tendency to spread than others. Sarcomas spread through the blood, often to the lung, liver, and brain	• Surgery • Radiation • Chemotherapy	Symptoms vary depending on the part of the body involved • Lumps • Pain • Fever • Weight loss • Fatigue

Skin Cancer: There are three main types of cells in the outer layer of skin: squamous cells, basal cells and melanocytes. Skin cancers are malignant lesions that occur in these cells.

Melanomas are related to the cells that make the pigment melanin. Skin cancers are generally associated with ultra violet light exposure. (Tiedemann 2009)

	Interventions	Commonly Experienced Symptoms
Basal and squamous cell cancers are less aggressive than malignant melanomas	• Surgical excision with wide margin • Regional lymph node dissection • Chemotherapy	• Change in size, shape, colour or diameter of an existing skin lesion • Appearance of a new lesion • Generally on sun exposed areas but can occur anywhere Melanoma: signs are promoted as ABCD • **A**symmetry-one half of the mole does not match the other half • **I**rregular border • **C**olour such as blue, black or variation in the same mole • **D**iameter greater than 6mm

Lymphomas are cancers of the B or T lymphocytes or natural killer cells that originate in the lymphatic system. There a two major categories, Hodgkin Lymphoma and non-Hodgkin Lymphomas. (Simpson 2009)		
Trajectory	Interventions	Commonly Experienced Symptoms
Hodgkin Lymphoma is considered a curable disease	• Chemotherapy • Immunotherapy • Radioimmunotherapy • Radiation therapy	• Unexplained weight loss • Unexplained fevers for more than 3 days • Drenching night sweats • Pruritis • Pain in involved areas after alcohol consumption • Painless adenopathy (cervical or supraclavicular) • Splenomegaly
Non Hodgkin Lymphomas		• Painless adenopathy (neck armpit, groin or abdomen • Fatigue • Pruritis MALT lymphoma affects the stomach lining and can cause nausea, vomiting and abdominal pain Cutaneous T-cell lymphoma affects the skin and cause raised patches, redness and itching

Dying Trajectories

Hallenbeck (2003) wrote that people desire, and also fear, certainty in life. They want to know what is going to happen, yet, when what is going to happen is not perceived as good, fear arises. A person who is informed that treatment is failing will often ask "How long do I have?" Perhaps having a time frame provides some sense of control for the dying person. For most serious and chronic disease processes, the quicker the decline, the sooner the death.

Reflecting on possible trajectories and applying that knowledge to each particular case can help formal caregivers to identify that a person is in the process of dying. Needs can be anticipated and supportive interventions initiated.

There are several ways of describing the dying process. Duration refers to the time involved between the onset of dying and the arrival of death. Shape refers to the course or the dying process for example, how predictable the process and timing will be (National Cancer Institute, 2005).

The following examples of dying trajectories related to cancer have been described:

1. The gradual slant trajectory is characterized by a long slow decline, sometimes lasting for years.

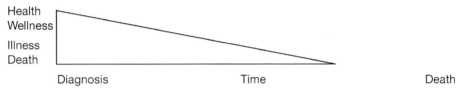

2. The steep downward slant trajectory is represented by a rapid decline toward death in which the chronic phase of the illness is either short or non existent.

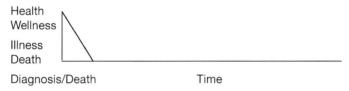

3. The peaks and valleys trajectory involves alternating periods of remission and relapse. Relapses tend to become more frequent as the illness progresses.

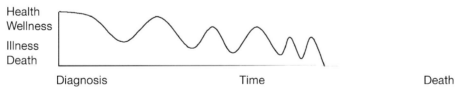

4. The descending plateaus trajectory, involves decline followed by restabilization. Each period of restabilization involves adjusting to a different level of functioning. The length of time the person remains in the stable phase tends to become shorter as the illness progresses.

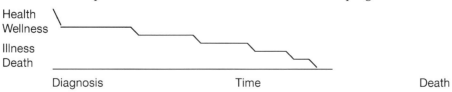

The following chart depicts another method used to describe dying trajectories and implications.

Trajectory	Description	Implications
Sudden Death	In this dying trajectory nothing can be done for the person found suddenly and unpredictably dead. Care of survivors is of paramount concern.	• Lack of preparation • No chance to say goodbye • Often no will, funeral plans • Bereavement needs are intense
Cancer Death	This dying trajectory, if recognized, offers the potential for getting one's house in order.	• Those with metastatic disease remain functional until about 5 to 6 months before death and then slowly decline until two to three months before death • Decline accelerates rapidly and symptom needs escalate • Individuals with advanced cancer who take to their beds without a correctable cause will usually die in a matter of weeks to months
Sine-Waving is a trajectory that involves oscillating or swinging back and forth from chronic ill health to acute crisis	This is the dying trajectory of congestive heart failure, chronic obstructive pulmonary disorder and many infirmities of advanced age. It involves periodic crises followed by stabilization. Any particular crisis could lead to death. If you would not be surprised if the person were to die in the next two years, the person has a serious life-limiting illness. Discussion and planning relative to end-of-life care is indicated.	• Health status is low for 6 to 24 months prior to death • Acute exacerbations occur intermittently and tend to increase over time • Frequent hospital admissions • Frequently not identified as dying • Live miserably on a roller coaster of decline and transient improvement
Death following Aggressive Life-Sustaining Treatment in Acute Care	This dying trajectory is common to many illnesses including chronic illnesses with sine-waving or those with acute catastrophic events such as stroke, overwhelming sepsis or adverse outcomes of surgery. Many will die as aggressive treatment continues.	• Enmeshed in high tech medicine • Probability of imminent death may not be recognized by individuals, families or staff. • Person doesn't die, the person "codes" • Emotional impact of death is great • Second thoughts and guilt arise
Predicted Death	Death will occur in the not too distant future, regardless of specific care decisions. When decision is made to withdraw high tech interventions, parties generally desire a quick death. The person who is on a ventilator and declared brain dead is an example of this trajectory.	• Shift or transition in the focus of care; decisions are related to withdrawal of treatment and the desired setting for the death to occur • Special communication skills are needed • Person and family may experience a sense of abandonment due to withdrawal of treatment • If death takes longer than expected, families who wish for the quick death may suffer intense guilt

Observing the Individual's Experience

Pain and other distressing symptoms can present in a number of ways. A variety of tools can assist with observing the presence and extent of symptoms.

The Edmonton Symptom Assessment System

One of the best ways to get an overall sense of how the person is experiencing his or her illness is to measure the burden of various physical, psychosocial, and spiritual symptoms. In order to facilitate a positive change in the experience of the illness, everything about the person's situation needs to be taken into consideration.

Since there can be significant differences in the perception of needs (e.g. between formal and informal caregiver, or caregivers and the person and family), the use of a validated tool to measure the burden of symptoms is helpful. The Edmonton Symptom Assessment System (ESAS) is a tool designed to assist in the assessment of a variety of symptoms and has been researched and validated with the cancer population (Bruera, Kuehn, Miller, Selmser, & Macmillan, 1991). Since all the symptoms on the tool have some relevance in other chronic illnesses and it is brief and easily administered, it can be easily applied in other diseases as well.

Early identification and reporting of symptoms may lead to improved management and better quality of life. The ESAS tool enables the person to identify the degree of distress/burden related to each particular symptom and helps us as caregivers to understand the impact of the disease on the person's quality of life. Caregivers can more readily engage in conversations related to goals of care when there is an understanding of the illness experience from the perspective of the person and family.

The ESAS was designed to allow the person or his or her family caregiver to self-administer the tool. It is the person's opinion of the severity of the symptoms that is the gold standard for symptom assessment.

The tool is designed to assist in the assessment of pain, tiredness, nausea, depression, anxiety, drowsiness, appetite, well being and shortness of breath. One "other problem" line is available for the person to use as needed. Since bowel function is a frequent symptom of those suffering with chronic illness, permission was sought to add bowel function to the list of symptoms and the tool with bowel function included is found in this resource guide. The severity at the time of the assessment of each symptom is rated from 0 – 10 on a numerical scale; with 0 meaning that the symptom is absent and 10 that it is the worst possible severity. The Edmonton Symptom Assessment System tool can be found online at http://www.cancercare.on.ca/toolbox/symptools/

The ESAS provides a clinical profile of symptom severity over time. Documentation of scores provides a context within which symptoms can begin to be understood. It is not a complete symptom assessment in itself. For good symptom management to be attained, the ESAS must be used as just one part of a holistic clinical assessment.

The ESAS tool was revised in 2010 based on results from research and years of use. The toll is now called ESAS-r to indicate the revised version.

Edmonton Symptom Assessment System (modified and revised) (ESAS-r)

Please circle the number that best describes how you feel NOW:

No pain	0 1 2 3 4 5 6 7 8 9 10	Worst possible pain

No tiredness *(Tiredness = lack of energy)* 0 1 2 3 4 5 6 7 8 9 10 Worst possible tiredness

Not drowsiness *(Drowsiness = feeling sleepy)* 0 1 2 3 4 5 6 7 8 9 10 Worst possible drowsiness

No nausea 0 1 2 3 4 5 6 7 8 9 10 Worst possible nausea

No lack of appetite 0 1 2 3 4 5 6 7 8 9 10 Worst possible lack of appetite

No shortness of breath 0 1 2 3 4 5 6 7 8 9 10 Worst possible shortness of breath

No depression *(Depression = feeling sad)* 0 1 2 3 4 5 6 7 8 9 10 Worst possible depression

No anxiety *(Anxiety = feeling nervous)* 0 1 2 3 4 5 6 7 8 9 10 Worst possible anxiety

Best wellbeing *(Wellbeing = how you feel overall)* 0 1 2 3 4 5 6 7 8 9 10 Worst possible wellbeing

Normal bowel function 0 1 2 3 4 5 6 7 8 9 10 Worst possible bowel function

No _____ other problem *(for example dry mouth)* 0 1 2 3 4 5 6 7 8 9 10 Worst Possible _____

Patient's Name _____

Date _____ Time _____

Complete by (check one)
- ◯ Patient
- ◯ Family Caregiver
- ◯ Health care professional caregiver
- ◯ Caregiver - assisted

Used and modified with permission, Regional Palliative Care Program, Edmonton Zone, Alberta Health Services, 2011.

BODY DIAGRAM ON FOLLOWING PAGE

Please mark on these pictures where it is you hurt.

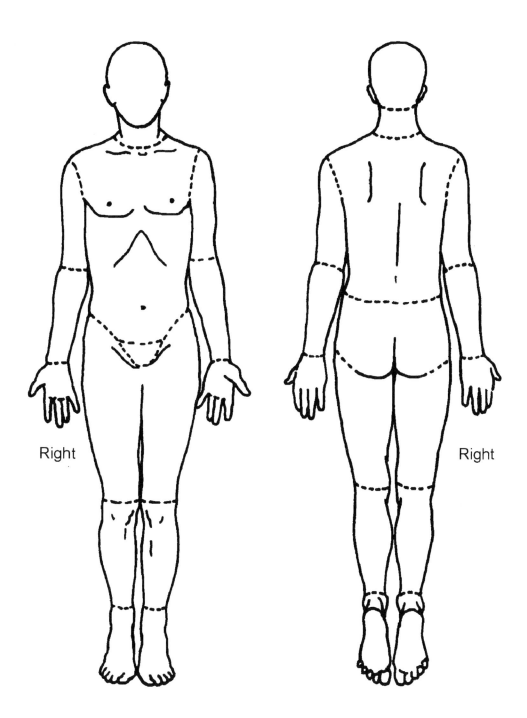

Right

Right

Completion of the ESAS-r

- The Regional Palliative Care Program of Edmonton, Alberta (2010) recommends the following when completing the ESAS-r:

- It is recommended that the person complete the ESAS-r *with guidance from a health care professional,* especially on the first occasion

- The person should be instructed to rate the severity of each symptom on a 0 to 10 scale, where 0 represents absence of the symptom and 10 represents the worst possible severity. The number should be circled on the scale

No pain   0   1   2   3   4   5   6   7   8   9   10   Worst possible pain

- The person should be instructed to rate each symptom according to how he or she feels *now*. The health care professional may choose to ask additional questions about the severity of symptoms at other time points e.g. symptom severity at best and at worst over the past 24 hours.

- *Definitions* have been added to items that have been found to be more problematic for people to understand or rate. You can review these with the person:

  Tiredness - lack of energy

  Drowsiness - feeling sleepy

  Depression - feeling sad

  Anxiety - feeling nervous

  Wellbeing - how you feel overall

- With the previous version of the ESAS, people often *reversed the scale for appetite* i.e. they considered "0" as "no appetite" and "10" as "best appetite". The scale has now been re-labeled as "lack of appetite". Coaching people on the correct direction of the scale is recommended

- The *body diagram* on the reverse side of the ESAS-r can be used to indicate sites of pain

- The circled numbers can be transcribed onto the ESAS-r graph

When to do the ESAS-r

- In palliative home care, complete and graph the ESAS-r during each telephone or personal contact. If symptoms are in good control, and there are no predominant psychosocial issues, then the ESAS-r can be completed weekly for people in the home.

- In hospice and tertiary palliative care units, the ESAS-r should be completed daily.

- In other settings, palliative care consultants will use the tool on initial assessments and follow up visits.

Who should do the ESAS-r

- Preference is for the person to provide the ratings of symptom severity

- If the person cannot provide ratings of severity but can provide input, then the ESAS-r is completed with help of a caregiver (family, friend, health professional involved in care)

- If the person cannot participate in the assessment at all or refuses to do so then this can be completed by the caregiver. Caregivers are encouraged to rate objectively

  Examples of objective indicators - grimacing and guarding for pain, increased time spent resting for tiredness, decreased level of alertness for drowsiness, retching or vomiting for nausea, quantity of food intake for appetite, increased respirations or effort causing distress for shortness of breath, tearfulness, flat affect, withdrawal for depression, agitation, flushing, restlessness for anxiety and how the person appears overall for well-being

- If it is not possible to rate a symptom, the caregiver may indicate "U" for "unable to assess"

- Indicate who completed the tool on the bottom of the ESAS-r.

Interacting with the Person and Formal/informal Caregivers

Communication with the person from the outset is important in building trust. If early symptoms of disease are dismissed and the person eventually is diagnosed with a serious disease, feelings of anger and frustration may affect the relationships with team members throughout the illness. If testing is prolonged, the person needs to be supported and encouraged to believe that an answer will come. The way in which the diagnosis is conveyed to the person will have an impact on how the person experiences the health care system. Awareness of the CLASS protocol (Buckman 2007) in all interactions is helpful in developing communication skills.

REMEMBER:
Context
Listening
Acknowledgement of emotion
Strategy for management
Summary

The health care provider needs to be mindful that his or her physical, emotional, or psychological exhaustion can affect the ability to communicate caring, empathy and compassion.

Therapeutic conversations with the person and family many involve the following:

- The seriousness of the illness

- The likely path the illness will take

- Goals, expectations, values and beliefs

- Treatment options including the benefits and burdens of various options.

Having a therapeutic conversation with the person and family may be challenging for some of the following reasons:

- Fear of upsetting a person by talking about his or her illness and dying

- Fear of extinguishing hope

- Fear of providing more information than expected/desired

- Fear of not having the right answers

- Lack of knowledge and skills around effective communication.

Health Care Team Sharing

What information will be helpful to team members in order to improve care?

- Understanding of the disease process and treatment goals (cure, prolonging life or palliation)

- Any particular concerns or wishes

- The Palliative Performance Scale score

- The understanding of the goals of treatment by both person and family

- The person's level of satisfaction related to the plan of treatment

- ESAS scores.

Person, Family and Friend Sharing

Often when the diagnosis of a life-threatening illness comes, friends and family will encourage positive thinking and discourage any reflection about death. They may give advice about any number of treatments that could result in cure and will promote the adoption of a "fighting spirit". It is not easy for the person with the illness, or his or her family and friends, to face the inevitable. Being realistic about the situation can be equated with giving up on the part of the person or lack of compassion and concern on the part of the caregiver.

Frequently, a person will only speak openly with those he or she has learned to trust and who have demonstrated understanding and good will. In some situations, a person may choose to confide in caregivers outside the family believing that the significant other is being spared the burden of a difficult conversation. Caregivers may be called upon to help break down barriers and end the silence by bringing family members together to discuss the illness, potential treatments, as well as the impending death. Acknowledging the "elephant" in the room is helpful but there are situations in which the person and / or family members will use denial as a coping mechanism until the very end of life.

Providing Supportive Care Strategies

The routes outlined in the "road map" for Navigating the Journey and the stages defined in the PPS (stable, transitional, and end-of-life), represent the progressive nature of life-threatening illnesses. Each person and family will have specific issues that need to be addressed along the illness trajectory.

A person waiting for test results may benefit from emotional support. The period of uncertainty while awaiting a diagnosis can be worse than receiving the diagnosis. Ambiguity generates anxiety. Determining the person's need for information and how he or she wishes to have news communicated gives the person a measure of control. When a diagnosis cannot be confirmed, acknowledging the ongoing search for answers can be supportive. Ensuring that the person has access to as much information as desired and is allowed to voice concerns is important. Symptom management, regardless of the fact that there is no diagnosis, is necessary to ensure the best possible quality of life.

Once a diagnosis is made, the person needs to be made aware of all the treatment options and determine which treatment options meet his or her goals. Appropriate information sharing related to the disease, treatment options and side effects is necessary for an informed consent. Throughout the journey with a life-threatening illness, the person and family continually face new challenges. An awareness of community resources, including support groups, empowers the person and family to access services that might be of benefit to them along the journey. It is often difficult for the person to attempt to cope with the demands of life while simultaneously attempting to comply with treatment and symptom management regimes and resulting side effects. Appropriate and early referrals to various team members will enhance comfort and support an enhanced quality of life for the person.

Throughout the illness trajectory, support in the face of changing treatment goals is necessary; even those who recover are often plagued with fear of disease recurrence.

The person and family may be searching and hoping for a cure and receive a variety of suggestions regarding alternative and/or complementary therapies. Because alternative treatments may have adverse interactions with prescribed treatments it is important for the caregiver to encourage the individual to inform his or her physician of all current therapies. Complementary therapies such as imagery, meditation, music and art can be very beneficial but care is required when using these therapies as powerful emotions can be released.

When it has been determined that there are no further curative options available for the person with a life-threatening illness, monitoring of PPS scores should be initiated. Cancer Care Ontario has developed three generic care plans that identify appropriate care interventions for each stage. The care plans are based on the domains of issues and the process of providing care from the model and address three stages that correspond to the Palliative Performance System Scores.

The Stable Stage Collaborative Care Plan is applicable for those with a PPS score between 100 % and 70%

The Transitional Stage Collaborative Care Plan is applicable for those with a PPS score between 60% and 40%.

The End of Life Collaborative Care Plan is applicable for those with a PPS score between 30 % and 0%.

The care plans can be found on the Cancer Care Ontario website; http://www.cancercare.on.ca/toolbox/pallcaretools/

The transition from PPS 20% to 10% is very different than other transitions; the families must make a critical shift from "doing" for the person to "being" with the person. Time spent with the person now shifts from predominantly task oriented activity to a quieter pace of sitting and providing companionship. Families start to focus on the time of death. (A Circle of Care: Victoria Hospice, 2001)

Working as a Team

Identifying and managing issues throughout the illness journey requires a team of caregivers whose members communicate consistently through the use of a common language and common tools. An integrated care plan with input from all disciplines ensures that everyone is on the same page and marching to the same drummer. The issues the person confronts and the symptoms identified and measured by the ESAS change throughout the illness journey. To ensure that the person's issues and distressing systems are managed and his or her wishes and goals are identified and incorporated into the care plan, the formal caregivers should consider the following:

- Know who the team members are at the different stages of the journey and how to get in contact with them

- Ensure that everyone is aware of the care plan whenever changes are made

- Communicate regularly to team members using standardized reporting format

- Implement comfort measures within each discipline's scope of practice and document the effectiveness of the measures

- Understand the PPS and communicate the score to the team

- Understand the ESAS and communicate the scores to the team

- Be aware of the challenge of working with many team members and the blending of roles

- Develop with the person a plan of care that addresses their goals for comfort and function and respects his/her rights

- Share a common knowledge base, tools and language for care planning and person/family education

- Respect each team member's contribution and role

Remember: The goal of care is to provide a combination of appropriate therapeutic interventions, agreed upon by the person, aimed at disease management, relieving suffering, and improving quality of life so as to facilitate a positive change of the experience of illness for the person and family.

Reference List

Alexandra, C. HIV/AIDS (2007) In L. Emmanuel & L. Librach (EDs). *Palliative Care Core Skills and Competencies*. Philadelphia: Saunders

Bruera, E., Kuehn, N., Miller, M., Selmser, P., and Macmillan, K. (1991). The Edmonton symptom assessment system (ESAS): A simple method for the assessment of palliative care patients. *Journal of Palliative Care*. 7:2. 6-9.

Buckman, R. (2007) Communication Skills. In L. Emmanuel & L. Librach (EDs). *Palliative Care Core Skills and Competencies*. Philadelphia: Saunders

Bunch, P. (2009) Gynecological Cancer. In S. Neuton, M. Hickey, J. Marrs (EDs). *Oncology Nursing Advisor A Comprehensive Guide to Clinical Practice*. St. Louis: Mosby

Collins, M., Bunch, P. (2009) Genitourinary Cancers. In S. Neuton, M. Hickey, J. Marrs (EDs). *Oncology Nursing Advisor A Comprehensive Guide to Clinical Practice*. St. Louis: Mosby

Edmonton Symptom Assessment System http://www.cancercare.on.ca/toolbox/symptools/

Egan, K. & Labyak, M. (2006). Hospice care: A model for quality end-of-life care. In B.R. Ferrell & N. Coyle (Eds.). *Textbook of palliative nursing*. New York: Oxford University Press.

Ferris, F.D., Balfour, H.M., Bowen, K., Farley, J., Hardwick, M., Lamontagne, C., Lundy, M., Syme, A., & West, P. (2002). *A model to guide hospice palliative care; Based on national principles and norms of practice*. Ottawa: Canadian Hospice Palliative Care Association.

Grande, C., Hoyer, K., Keith, B., Agbajani, B., Smith-Zamiska, M., Roll, M. (2009) Gastrointestinal System. In S. Neuton, M. Hickey, J. Marrs (EDs). *Oncology Nursing Advisor A Comprehensive Guide to Clinical Practice*. St. Louis: Mosby

Groninger, J., Muir, J. (2007) Pulmonary Palliative Medicine. In L. Emmanuel & L. Librach (EDs). *Palliative Care Core Skills and Competencies*. Philadelphia: Saunders

Hallenbeck, J. (2003) *Palliative Care Perspectives*. New York: Oxford University Press.

Hauser, J., Bonow, R. (2007) Heart Disease. In Emmanuel, L. & Librach, L. (EDs). *Palliative Care Core Skills and Competencies*. Philadelphia: Saunders

Jones, C., Coleman, S. (2007) Neurodegenerative Diseases. In L. Emmanuel & L. Librach (EDs). *Palliative Care Core Skills and Competencies*. Philadelphia: Saunders

Klemm, P., Hurst, M. (2009) Cancer Pathophysiology. In S. Neuton, M. Hickey, J. Marrs (EDs). *Oncology Nursing Advisor A Comprehensive Guide to Clinical Practice*. St. Louis: Mosby

Leaby, N., Fortenbaugh, C. (2009) Sarcomas. In S. Neuton, M. Hickey, J. Marrs (EDs). *Oncology Nursing Advisor A Comprehensive Guide to Clinical Practice*. St. Louis: Mosby

Modi, S., KApo, J., Casarett, D. (2007) Chronic Diseases and Geriatrics. In L. Emmanuel & L. Librach (EDs). *Palliative Care Core Skills and Competencies*. Philadelphia: Saunders

Moss, A. (2007) Kidney Failure. In L. Emmanuel & L. Librach (EDs). *Palliative Care Core Skills and Competencies*. Philadelphia: Saunders

Page, M., Fedoroff, A. (2009) Central Nervous System. In S. Neuton, M. Hickey, J. Marrs (EDs). *Oncology Nursing Advisor A Comprehensive Guide to Clinical Practice*. St. Louis: Mosby

Payne, Y. (2009) Breast Cancer. In S. Neuton, M. Hickey, J. Marrs (EDs). *Oncology Nursing Advisor A Comprehensive Guide to Clinical Practice*. St. Louis: Mosby

Simpson, J. (2009) The Leukemias. In S. Neuton, M. Hickey, J. Marrs (EDs). *Oncology Nursing Advisor A Comprehensive Guide to Clinical Practice*. St. Louis: Mosby

Simpson, J. (2009) The Lymphomas. In S. Neuton, M. Hickey, J. Marrs (EDs). *Oncology Nursing Advisor A Comprehensive Guide to Clinical Practice*. St. Louis: Mosby

Simpson, J. (2009) Multiple Myloma. In S. Neuton, M. Hickey, J. Marrs (EDs). *Oncology Nursing Advisor A Comprehensive Guide to Clinical Practice.* St. Louis: Mosby

Strobl, R. (2009) Head and Neck Cancers. In S. Neuton, M. Hickey, J. Marrs (EDs). *Oncology Nursing Advisor A Comprehensive Guide to Clinical Practice.* St. Louis: Mosby

Tiedemann, D. (2009) Lung Cancer. In S. Neuton, M. Hickey, J. Marrs (EDs). *Oncology Nursing Advisor A Comprehensive Guide to Clinical Practice.* St. Louis: Mosby

Tiedemann, D. (2009) Skin Cancer. In S. Neuton, M. Hickey, J. Marrs (EDs). *Oncology Nursing Advisor A Comprehensive Guide to Clinical Practice.* St. Louis: Mosby

University of Maryland (2008) Liver Disease. Retrieved from http://www.umm.edu/liver/chronic.htm February 2011

Chapter Four

Domain: Physical

Physical

- Pain and other symptoms
- Level of consciousness, cognition
- Function, safety, aids (motor, senses, physiologic, sexual)
- Fluids, nutrition
- Wounds
- Habits

Person and Family

- Demographics
- Culture
- Personal values, beliefs, practices and strengths
- Developmental stage, education, literacy
- Disabilities

Ferris et al., 2002

Understanding the Fundamentals

Depending on the disease process, a person can experience a variety of physical symptoms such as pain, vomiting, shortness of breath, constipation, and fatigue. Often, as the illness progresses, the person experiences not only one but several issues and physical symptoms on a daily basis. The combination of issues and symptoms greatly impacts the person's quality of life.

Consider the person living with advanced bone cancer, experiencing severe back pain increasing in intensity with every movement, unable to sleep or eat due to nausea, constipated from medications, fatigued, depressed, feeling isolated and concerned about being a burden to his or her family. That's an example of a person experiencing distressing issues in several domains. Profound suffering can be the result of a single distressing issue or a combination of symptoms and circumstances that impact wellbeing.

The term Total Pain was coined by Dame Cicely Saunders, a nurse, social worker and physician and the founder of the modern hospice movement. Complex and multiple issues in all the domains of issues associated with the illness and bereavement; disease management, physical, psychological, social, spiritual, practical, end-of-life care/death management, and loss and grief account for a condition called TOTAL PAIN. Pain does not occur in isolation; it affects all those who are in contact with the person. Balfour Mount (2007) speaks of the noble task of caring for the seriously ill person and his or her family with "tough clinical science and compassion". That was Dame Cicely's challenge to those of us working in hospice palliative care. Management of total pain calls for integrated care plans that reach for perfection in terms of managing physical symptoms and psychosocial and spiritual suffering. The process of dying seems to act as a catalyst in setting free the innate healing potential which resides in each individual. Skilled health care providers need to remember that quality of life is not dependant on the management of physical issues alone but with good pain and symptom control, an environment can be created in which healing at a deep personal level can occur. Mount (2007) in Emmanuel and Librach

The figure below portrays the fact that the person who is living with life-limiting illness is frequently bombarded with issues from every direction and deep suffering or total pain results. Examples of issues from each domain that create the suffering follow.

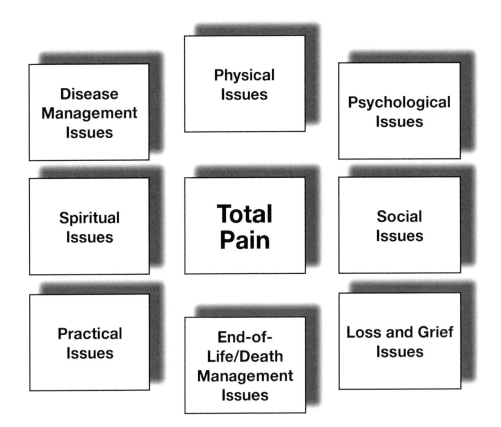

Total Pain

1. Disease Management

- Concern about advancing illness,
- Concern about adverse effects from medications/treatments
- Concern about existing conditions and allergies.

2. Physical

- Unmanaged pain
- Unmanaged symptoms; nausea, shortness of breath, constipation, etc
- Sleep disturbances
- Increasing fatigue, diminishing appetite, diminishing strength and mobility.

3. Psychological

- Emotions associated with increasing losses; loss of role, loss of dignity, loss of control/independence/autonomy
- Compromised self image
- Increasing anxiety related to anticipated decline in health status and the dying process
- Concern about unpredictable flood of emotions; anger, sadness, fear.

4. Social

- Diminishing role within the family, workplace, community
- Changing family relationships, compromised intimacy
- Diminishing social routines/relationships
- Concern about becoming a burden
- Feelings of isolation and abandonment
- Concerns about finances, housing, property, wills.

5. Spiritual

- Struggle to find meaning and purpose in life
- Increasing feelings of hopelessness
- Questioning and re-evaluating religious beliefs
- Feelings of guilt and regret.

6. Practical

- Diminishing ability to perform ADL's and IADL's such as driving, shopping, and communicating by telephone, email, etc.
- Concern about increasing caregiver burden
- Concern about pets and home maintenance.

7. End-of-Life Care/Death Management

- Fear of the unknown
- Fear of increasing pain and symptoms and that distress will not be managed
- Fear of the dying process
- Fear of abandonment
- Fear of indignity to the body after death.

8. Loss, Grief

- "Struggle to let go"
- Grief related to loss of sense of self as a person, loss of roles, diminishing prestige and ultimately the separation of body and spirit at the time of death
- Grief related to loss of relationships, particularly those most cherished
- Grief related to the inability to participate in future events such as the graduation or wedding of a child
- Grief related to loss of income, home, possessions, treasures.

In this chapter that deals with issues in the physical domain, we will address the common symptoms of physical pain, dyspnea and constipation. There are numerous other physical symptoms that impact the well-being of those with progressive illness but these three will be dealt with in more detail.

Pain

Fink and Gates (2006) note that "pain is a common companion of birth, growth, death and illness; it is intertwined intimately with the very nature of human existence". Few things are of more concern to the person and family at end-of-life than the control of pain. However, people should not have to live their lives in pain waiting for the end of life to have health care providers and caregivers address their pain. An understanding of pain by all formal and informal caregivers is of utmost importance. We must all advocate for pain relief whenever it is identified.

A variety of definitions exist for pain:

- McCaffery and Pasero (1999) define pain as being whatever the experiencing person says it is, existing whenever the experiencing person says it does
- RNAO (2007) states that pain is subjective (occurring where and when the person indicates it does), multidimensional and a highly variable experience for everyone regardless of age or special needs
- Thai and Fainsinger (2007) define pain as a biopsychosocial event
- The International Association for the Study of Pain (2007) defines pain as "an unpleasant sensory and emotional experience associated with actual or potential tissue damage, or described in terms of such damage".

Types of Pain

There are two categories of pain – acute and chronic. Acute pain is associated with tissue damage, inflammation, a disease process that is relatively short or a surgical procedure. Acute pain warns the person that something is wrong. Chronic pain on the other hand is persistent, worsens over time, and endures for an extended period of time and results in decreased function and well-being. Chronic pain is further divided into malignant pain and non-malignant pain. Regardless of the type of pain, all pain should be addressed with the same rapid and comprehensive management approach. Remember: "Pain is whatever the person says and occurs whenever the person says it does" (McCaffery, 1999).

Acute Pain	
Characteristics	Responses
• Recent onset • Transient in nature • Lasts for a limited time (several minutes to several days, usually under 30 days) • Usually caused by tissue damage • Associated with some degree of inflammation	• May be anxiety depending on the intensity, predictability and meaning of the pain • May be overt pain behaviours e.g. grimacing, splinting, • Sympathetic nervous system signs e.g. increased pulse and respiration rates, sweating, raised BP

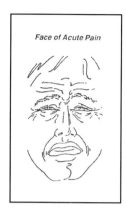

Face of Acute Pain

Chronic or Persistent Pain	
Characteristics	Responses
• Persists beyond the usual course of an injury or disease resolution; usually beyond 3 to 6 months. • Pattern of recurrence over months or years • Associated with a chronic pathological condition	• Emotional, depressive symptoms e.g. isolation, anxiety, guilt, fatigue, sadness • Objective physiological signs are often absent

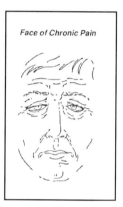

Face of Chronic Pain

The face of acute pain and the face of chronic pain reproduced from Cancer Pain: A Monograph on the Management of Cancer (1984). Health and Welfare Canada. The characteristics and responses to acute and chronic or persistent pain are derived from Jovey (2008).

The American Geriatric Society (Fink and Gates 2010) has classified chronic or persistent pain into subcategories in order to assist the care provider to determine the best management strategy based on the subtype. These include:

1. Nociceptive pain resulting from stimulation of peripheral pain receptors
   a. Visceral: pain associated with organs such as lungs, liver, heart etc.
   b. Somatic: superficial somatic pain (skin) and deep somatic pain (bone, muscle, ligaments, joints)

2. Neuropathic pain resulting from peripheral or central nervous system stimulation

3. Mixed or unspecified pain

4. Pain due to psychological disorders

Pain can be categorized using other terms as well.

1. Anticipatory Pain
   • Having experienced pain in a certain situation, the person expects to have pain in a similar circumstance
   • Has the effect of causing fear and anxiety

2. Baseline Pain
   • A constant pain state for at least half of the day

3. Breakthrough Pain
   - A transitory increase in pain over and above baseline pain
   - Causes increased psychological distress and significant decreases in function

4. Incident Pain
   - A type of breakthrough pain
   - Results from movement or action
     (e.g. turning in bed, sitting to standing, painful dressing changes)

5. Remembered Pain
   - Usually never forgotten
   - Certain events or times of day can trigger it

Components of the Pain Experience

Many components may drive the person's response to pain and his or her willingness to accept certain care strategies. Understanding these components will help in the provision of more individualized pain management strategies. There will always be unique expressions of pain. Information in the following chart was gathered from Al-Atiyyat, (2009) and McCaffery and Pasero (1999).

Component	Description	Example
Cultural Background	Individuals will react to pain in the manner they have learned as acceptable within their group.	If the family values "stoicism" the person will be silent If the family values pathos, there will be behavioural indications e.g. crying, moaning etc
Gender	A society's attitudes can influence the way a male should respond and react to pain versus how a female should respond and react to pain	A woman may be allowed to cry Men are expected to not cry
Age	With increasing age, tolerance to cutaneous pain increases and tolerance to deep pain decreases.	Reporting of pain by the elderly may differ from that of younger persons and they may be more stoic about pain. Differences among age and gender maybe the result of older females tending to carry on ethnic traditions more than younger males
Meaning of pain	Pain is determined by the interpretation of what the pain means to the person	Person may perceive increased pain to be related to worsening disease. Some people may interpret pain as a punishment for past sins. Some people do not see pain as evil or negative but part of life
Life experiences	An individual's previous experiences with pain will influence how he or she responds to pain	Repeated experiences with pain usually teach the person how severe pain can become and how difficult it is to get relief. Such persons may have higher levels of anxiety and lower pain threshold

Pain Threshold

Pain Threshold is defined as that point at which the individual feels an increasing intensity of stimuli as painful. Everyone does not perceive the same intensity of pain from the same stimuli (McCaffery & Pasero, 1999). A person's pain threshold can be raised or lowered based on several factors. A chart with examples follows.

Factors that Raise Pain Threshold	Factors that Lower Pain Threshold
• Relief of symptoms • Sleep • Rest • Sympathy and understanding • Companionship • Diversional activity • Elevation of mood • Anti-depressants • Anxiolytics • Analgesics	• Discomfort • Insomnia • Fatigue • Anxiety • Fear • Sadness • Depression • Boredom • Introversion • Social isolation

There are many different causes and effects of pain; the following chart highlights some of the most common.

Causes of Pain	Effects of Pain
• **Arthritis:** low back pain, painful peripheral joints, especially hips, shoulders, knees • **Musculo-skeletal:** compression fractures of the spine, old hip and other fractures, contractures • **Diabetes:** peripheral neuropathy • **Cancer:** bone infiltration, nerve compression, raised intra-cranial pressure, therapy related to the disease, soft tissue damage • **Cardio-vascular:** angina, claudication, CVA • **Muscle spasm** • **Constipation:** rectal pressure, urinary incontinence, confusion, abdominal cramps, and diarrhea • **Oral Pain:** poorly fitting dentures, decayed teeth, gum disease, candidiasis • **Soft Tissue:** bruises, skin tears • **Visceral damage:** ulcerative colitis, tumour • **Ulceration:** decubitus ulcers • **Lymphedema:** swelling of limbs due to congestive heart disease, cancer • **Herpetic neuralgia:** related to "shingles"	**Physical** • Decreased functional capability • Poor appetite, interrupted sleep • Diminished strength/endurance • Increased constipation • Reduced activities of daily living **Psychological** • Diminished leisure, enjoyment • Increased fear, anxiety, anger • Depression • Loss of control • Resistance to care • Self abuse • Distressful and difficult behaviour **Social** • Diminished social relationship • Decreased sexual function • Increased caregiver burden • Distraught families • Isolation and decreased quality of life **Spiritual** • Increased suffering; "why is this happening to me?" • Re-evaluation of religious beliefs • Demoralization

Barriers to Optimal Pain Assessment and Management

Some common barriers to effective pain assessment and management have been identified by Fink and Gates (2010) under the three headings that follow.

1. Person / Family / Societal Barriers

- The subjective and personal nature of the pain experience
- Lack of awareness on the part of person and family regarding pain assessment
- Lack of communication with health care professionals about pain
  - Reluctance to report pain
  - Not wanting to bother staff
  - Fear of not being believed
  - Stoicism
  - What's the use; nothing works
  - Concern that curative therapy might be curtailed if pain and symptom management become a focus.
- Lack of common language to describe pain
- Unfounded beliefs, misconceptions, and myths about pain and its treatment
  - Pain is inevitable
  - If pain is worse, the disease is spreading
  - Should wait to take medication until it is really needed
  - Too much medication now means there will nothing for later
  - Family think I am too 'spacey" so better cut back
  - If it's morphine, I must be close to the end
  - Taking medication will lead to addiction
  - If the medication is taken before it really hurts, I'll get too much
  - Best to hang in, just tough it out
  - I'd rather not be constipated
  - Don't want to bother the staff; they are busy with other people
  - Too much pain medication will hasten death
  - Good patients don't complain.

2. Health Care Professional Barriers

- Prejudice and bias; not believing the person; paternalistic attitudes
- Lack of identification of pain, pain assessment, and relief as a priority in patient care
- Inadequate knowledge about how to perform a pain assessment
- Perceived lack of time for pain assessments
- Failure to use validated tools
- Inability of clinician to empathize or establish rapport
- Concern about addiction
- Confusion related to addiction, tolerance and physical dependence
- Poor understanding of opioid side effects
- Low expectation for successful pain management
- Lack of consultation with secondary experts
- Cultural attitudes and beliefs
- Confusion around ethical and moral principles
- Fear of being accused of practising euthanasia, hurrying death.

3. System Barriers

- A system that fails to hold staff accountable for pain assessment and management
- Lack of tools for pain assessment and management in the setting
- Lack of institutional policies for performance and documentation of pain assessment
- Misinterpretation of stringent laws inhibits the appropriate use of opioids
- Confusion between the legitimate and illegitimate use of opioids
- Focus on cure rather than care
- Lack of co-ordination as people move through the system
- Red tape involved to obtain analgesics not normally covered by government plan.

Of the barriers to effective pain management previously listed, two of the most persistent barriers to pain management are myths about pain and myths about opioids.

Common Myths About Pain and Opioids

Myth: *Pain is a normal part of aging.*

Fact: Pain is a result of disease process or injury. Pain is not synonymous with aging.

Myth: *Pain is only felt while one is awake.*

Fact: Pain can be experienced while sleeping, hence the need for around-the-clock dosing.

Myth: *Pain can only be controlled with strong opioids.*

Fact: While opioids are frequently used to control pain, non-opioid medications and non-drug therapies can also be helpful.

Myth: *Opioids make you feel high.*

Fact: Pain management may make the person feel better but getting a high is uncommon.

Myth: *Opioids cause respiratory depression which can lead to death.*

Fact: When opioids are utilized for pain management and are properly titrated, respiratory depression is virtually non-existent.

Myth: *Opioids cause addiction.*

Fact: Addiction is very uncommon when opioids are utilized properly for pain management.

Myth: *Persons on opioids develop tolerance and over time the medications won't work anymore.*

Fact: Tolerance is a factor with long-term use of opioids but is not necessarily the reason for upward titration. There is no ceiling dose.

Myth: *"Shots" are stronger than pills*

Fact: Oral route is effective and preferred.

One of the biggest barriers to the more effective use of opioids to treat pain is the fear of causing addiction. In order to understand the management of pain and other symptoms common in hospice palliative care it is important to be familiar with the body and brain's response to medication when it is used as part of a treatment strategy. There are a number of terms used to differentiate these responses. (Jovey 2008)

1. Addiction

- A primary, chronic neurobiological disease, with genetic, psychosocial, and environmental factors, influencing its development and manifestations. It is characterized by behaviours that include one or more of the following (4**C**s)
  - Impaired **C**ontrol over drug use
    - May be reflected in requests for early prescription refills, double doctoring, using street sources
  - **C**ompulsive use
    - May be reflected in non-compliance with non-opioid components of the plan, inability to acknowledge psychosocial contributors to pain, or the perception that nothing but opioids will relieve the pain.
  - **C**ontinued use despite harm or **C**onsequences
    - Consequences associated with use of opioids may include persistent over sedation or euphoria, deteriorating level of function despite pain relief, increased distress such as anxiety, sleep disturbance or depression.
  - **C**raving
    - Manifested as an intense desire to use a substance for its psychoactive effect rather than for the analgesic effect or to stave off physiological withdrawal symptoms.

2. Pseudo-Addiction

- A phenomenon in which those with severe, unrelieved pain may become intensely focused on finding relief for pain.
  - A behavioural process that mimics psychological dependence; this behaviour is related to poor pain management; the person has a "pain relief" seeking behaviour versus a "drug seeking" behaviour.

3. Tolerance

- A state of adaptation in which exposure to a drug induces changes that result in a diminution of one or more of the drug's effects over time
  - Tolerance to most of the unwanted opioid side (nausea, sedation, respiratory depression) effects occurs rapidly
  - Tolerance to the analgesic effects is indicated by the need for increasing or more frequent doses of the medication to maintain the analgesic effect
  - Occurs in an area of the brain separate from the brain pathways related to addiction.

4. Physical Dependence

- A state of adaptation that often includes tolerance and is manifested by a drug class-specific withdrawal syndrome that can be produced by abrupt cessation, rapid dose reduction, decreasing blood level of the drug and / or administration of an antagonist.
  - Expected physiological response
  - May develop in 7-10 days
  - Occurs in an area of the brain thought to be unrelated to addiction.

Dyspnea

Dyspnea is a frequently encountered symptom in progressive life-limiting illness and it may be just as distressing as pain, or more so, to the person and his or her family. Shortness of breath requires as aggressive assessment and management as pain. Remember that opioids are indicated for dyspnea as well as for pain.

The American Thoracic Society defines dyspnea as "the term used to characterize a subjective experience of breathing discomfort that consists of qualitatively distinct sensations that vary in intensity."(Dudgeon 2011)

The experience derives from interactions among multiple physiological, psychological, social and environmental factors, and may induce secondary physiological and behavioral responses.

More simply stated, dyspnea is an uncomfortable awareness of breathing and is associated with:
- functional and social limitations
- suffering
- psychological distress
- impaired quality of life.

Dyspnea is often present for long periods of time in the illness trajectory of many progressive diseases. Dudgeon (2006) notes that dyspnea is reported to be an issue for 50% of cancer outpatients with the incidence rising to 70% in the terminal phase of the disease. Shortness of breath is a distressing symptom for approximately 90% of those with lung cancer. Persons with end stage COPD (95%) report extreme breathlessness. Over half the individuals with CHF have found dyspnea to be a major concern in the last year of life. Dyspnea is also reported by persons with ALS, dementia and stroke. The presence of dyspnea accounts for 25 to 53% cases in which palliative sedation is required for uncontrolled symptoms. (Shroder and Dudgeon 2007) Those with dyspnea are more likely to die in hospital than at home partly due to the increased distress for caregivers and staff. Unfortunately, doctors and nurses do not always provide proper assistance and leave the person and family to cope with this debilitating symptom in isolation. Like pain, dyspnea is a subjective symptom and *it is what the person says it is.* When asking about shortness of breath it is important to ask about the person's experience at rest, while walking, climbing stairs or eating. Reports of dyspnea must be taken seriously by the team and every effort made to alleviate this symptom.

Constipation

Constipation is another symptom that causes untold distress for many persons with debilitating illness or using medications such as opioids to relieve pain or dyspnea. Constipation is common, affecting 70 to 100% of cancer patients, and yet undertreated by both physicians and nurses. (Economou 2006) Constipation causes physical, social and psychological distress and affects quality of life. Proactive anticipation and management of constipation will prevent the difficulties encountered in relieving the problem. Nurses need to monitor bowel function on an ongoing basis throughout the illness trajectory. All health care providers need to take complaints of constipation seriously and address the problem immediately beginning with a proper assessment. The Victoria Bowel Performance Scale and Bowel Management Guidelines can be downloaded from the following web site: www.victoriahospice.org/health-professionals.../clinical-tools

Other Physical Symptoms

Some physical symptoms other than pain, dyspnea and constipation are listed below. This list is not exhaustive and the person can experience any number of symptoms.

- Anorexia/ loss of appetite
- Bleeding
- Cough
- Confusion

- Diarrhea
- Dysphagia (difficulty swallowing)
- Seizures
- Weakness

- Hiccoughing
- Sweating
- Nausea/vomiting
- Pruritis (itching)
- Insomnia

- Wounds
- Urinary frequency and/or Incontinence
- Urinary retention

Reflecting on the person's situation (pain or other symptoms) with the question "Why does this person have this symptom now?" initiates the gathering of data as part of the assessment required in order to determine an effective management plan.

Observing the Individual's Experience

Identifying the person's physical symptoms is critical in order to facilitate a change in the illness experience for the person and family. In order to address symptoms, the caregiver must understand the individual's experience - an understanding that is gained through knowledge of the disease process, careful observation and active listening.

Observing Pain

McCaffery & Pasero, (1999) suggest that there is an "order of importance" related to pain intensity that professionals should bear in mind when considering pain.

- Person's self-report using a pain rating scale e.g. the ESAS tool is the best indicator
- Pathologic conditions or procedures that usually cause pain should alert professionals to observe for signs of pain
- Behaviours (e.g., facial expressions, body movements, crying) are frequently seen in those with cognitive impairment and those who cannot verbally express pain
- Reports of pain from family or others close to the person can assist professionals in understanding how pain will be expressed or why it will not be expressed
- Physiologic measures such as B/P or pulse are the least sensitive indicators of pain.

The following indicators of pain are particularly important in identifying pain in a non verbal person e.g. cognitively impaired adults, infants and young children. There are a number of assessment tools that can be utilized in this population.

1. A change in facial expression.
   - A pained facial expression most often reflects the presence of physical pain (from usually relaxed to continuously troubled with wrinkled forehead, frowning, wide open or 'scrunched' eyes with distressed look).

2. A change in behaviour
   - Behaviours that indicate distress may reflect physical, intellectual, emotional, environmental, spiritual, or psychosocial pain. (P.I.E.C.E.S., 2011) A caregiver may observe any of the following behaviour changes:
     - from being quiet, still to moaning, rocking
     - from being friendly, outgoing to being combative, resisting care
     - from being involved in activities to being withdrawn
     - from cheerful to sad, crying easily
     - from eating well to refusing food
     - from sleeping well to being awake much of the night.
   - A new behaviour or change in gestures such as wringing of the hands, fidgeting with clothes, "pleating", clenching fists, resisting care, holding onto the chair as though needing security.
   - A change in body movements such as tossing and turning in bed, flinging the arms about, reflexive jerking away, rubbing a body part, rhythmic body movements (e.g. banging on a table).
   - A change in posture such as slouching or a slow shuffling gait (suggests dejection or physical discomfort), tense posture and a rapid determined gait (suggest anxiety and/or anger), tense sitting and lying positions.

When family/staff/volunteers report a suspicion of pain further investigation should take place. Any change in the person's condition should warrant an inquiry about pain. Pain as the 5th vital sign is a concept that is being advocated in many settings. Whenever temperature, BP, pulse and respirations are taken, the person should be asked to rate pain as well. When a condition which is normally associated with pain is diagnosed, providers need to monitor for pain. When provided with information that the person is stoic and will not acknowledge pain the caregivers need to use different terminology to illicit information e.g. discomfort, soreness, uncomfortable.

When it has been determined that pain is an issue for the person, it is important that a pain assessment be completed to collect as much information as possible concerning the pain. A thorough assessment and a pain diagnosis are the key to an effective management plan. Pain assessment and monitoring forms have been developed to facilitate consistency in reporting. The RNAO Best Practice Guidelines for the Assessment and Management of Pain (2007) provides samples of tools used for pain assessment. Further information is available at www.rnao.org.

As part of the initial pain assessment as well as the ongoing monitoring of pain, it is important to attempt to quantify the pain a person is experiencing. The most commonly used scales that have proven to be effective in measuring pain are (Fink & Gates, 2010):

1. The Visual Analogue Scale (VAS)
2. The Numeric Rating Scale (NRS)
3. Verbal Descriptor Scale (VDS)
4. Faces Scale (Wong-Baker)
5. The Faces Pain Scale Revised (FPS-R)
6. Pain Thermometer

See **Appendix A** *for a visual of the various pain intensity scales.*

The Edmonton Symptom Assessment System that is advocated for use throughout Ontario by Cancer Care Ontario uses a numeric rating scale for a number of commonly experienced symptoms related to chronic progressive illnesses. The tool is one of the best ways to get an overall sense of how the person is experiencing his or her illness. The tool measures the burden of various symptoms that together have a significant effect on the person's overall sense of wellbeing. In order to facilitate a positive change in the experience of the illness, everything about the person's situation needs to be taken into consideration.

Observing Dyspnea

As with pain, the person's self report is the most accurate indicator of the level of distress. Observations of the following should be made when dyspnea is an issue.

- Skin tone and colour
- Use of accessory muscles
- Pursed lips
- Ability to speak
- Positioning e.g. seated leaning forward
- Agitation and restlessness
- Mood, ability to concentrate and solve problems
- Level of distress related to walking, going shopping, making a bed
- Respiratory rate

Remember that an abnormally fast or slow rate of respiration is not necessarily indicative of a subjective experience of shortness of breath.

There are a number of tools that can be used to measure dyspnea; the Visual Analog Scale, the Oxygen Cost Diagram, the Modified Borg Scale, Reading Numbers Aloud Test and the ESAS which is a numeric scale.

Observing Constipation

Besides observing the frequency, amount and consistency of stool other symptoms associated with constipation such as abdominal distension or bloating, change in amount of gas passed rectally, oozing of liquid stool, rectal fullness or pressure, rectal pain with bowel movements, and degree of strain required to pass stool should be noted. There are a number of tools available for assessment and management of constipation e.g. The Constipation Assessment Scale and the Victoria Hospice Bowel Performance Scale.

Interacting with the Individual and Formal/Informal Caregivers

Each person's symptom experience is unique. The person's past experiences with pain and other symptoms, progression of illness, cognition, culture, and many other factors affect the ability and willingness to communicate the experience.

Failure to believe the person's report of pain and/ or other physical symptoms may result in potentially harmful effects such as failing to detect a complication or to provide adequate treatment. Using a tool as a guide can help the novice clinician to gain all of the important information but usually a few questions such as "Tell me about your pain/ symptom? or "Describe how your pain/symptom is affecting your life?" will bring forth a great deal of information that can be documented on the tool without having to ask too many questions. Through active listening and clarifying, the clinician can usually gain most of the answers needed. The report of the person's word descriptors related to pain or other symptoms is crucial. Such descriptions are particularly important in diagnosing the type of pain and implementing the appropriate interventions. Any barriers, misunderstandings or myths must be uncovered if compliance with the plan of treatment is to be expected. It may take many consistent explanations from all the members of the team in order to convince the person of the wisdom of the plan. Identification and communication of the goals of the person and family with regard to pain and symptom management is paramount. If goals are not being met with the current treatment plan, health care providers have a duty to advocate for consultations with secondary of tertiary level experts in the field. Nurses are legally and ethically obligated to advocate for persons within the health care system to ensure that the most effective pain relieving strategies are utilized in promoting the person's comfort and the relief of pain (RNAO, 2007).

Providing Supportive Care Strategies

Much of hospice palliative care revolves around management of pain and other symptoms. There is nothing a care provider can do for a person that is more important to the experience of the illness than the management of symptoms resulting from his or her disease or its treatment. The traditional health care system utilizes medications and other treatments such as, chemotherapy, radiation, Trans Electrical Nerve Stimulation, heat, cold, acupuncture etc to manage physical pain. Individuals can choose other modalities as well. Most are on a fee for service basis. A discussion of alternative and complementary therapies follows.

Complementary Therapies

In recent years there has been a growing interest in Complementary Therapies. In this program, the term Complementary Therapies is used rather than Alternative Therapies. The distinction is important:

1. Alternative Therapy

   • Choice between one or another therapy; one is chosen to the exclusion of others.

2. Complementary Therapy

   • That which completes or supplies a deficiency

   • Adds the psychosocial and spiritual component to a holistic care approach

   • Many of these therapies open the person's spirit to experiences that transcend the pain of the present experience and provide insight, comfort, peace, and meaning.

Complementary Therapies include: (list retrieved from the RNAO Complementary Therapies Nursing Interest Group February 2011)

Acupressure	Acupuncture	Affirmations
Alexander Method	Aromatherapy	Art Therapy
Ayurvedic Medicine	Bach Flower Remedies	Bioenergetics
Biofeedback	Body Toning	Bowen Therapy
Chakra Balancing	Craniosacral Therapy	Colonhydrotherapy
Expressive Arts Therapies	Dream Interpretation	Feldenkrais
Facial Therapy	Herbalist	Healing Touch
Hypnosis	Homeopathy	Visualization
Imagery	Kinesiology	Iris Analysis
Light Touch Therapy	Labyrinth	Meditation
Massage Therapy	Moxibustion (Cupping)	Mitzvah Technique
Music Therapy	Naturopathy	Nutrition
Neuro-Linguistic Programming	Osteopathy	Pilates
Polarity Therapy	Prayer	Reiki
Reflexology	Rolfing	Shiatsu
Spiritual Healing	Tai Chi	Therapeutic Touch
Traditional/ Shamanic Healing	Trager Approach	Yoga

Supportive Strategies for Pain

- Believe the person
- Conduct a thorough assessment
- Implement the treatment plan consented to by the person
  - Pharmacological: non-opioid analgesics, opioids, adjuvant medications such as corticosteroids, tricyclic antidespressants, anticonvulsants, bisphospinates, muscle relaxants, anaesthetic agents
  - Non pharmacholgical: distraction, radiation therapy, relaxation therapy, physical and occupational therapy, TENS, acupuncture, heat, cold, other complementary therapies
- Monitor effectiveness of interventions
- Consult with experts if goals are not met within a predetermined time period(e.g. 48 hrs).

Supportive Strategies for Dyspnea

- Conduct a thorough assessment
- Implement the treatment plan consented to by the person.
- Administer opioids, bronchodilators, anxiolytics, oxygen as directed
- Be calm and reassuring
- Position: sitting up and leaning forward supporting arms on a table
- Educate person and family; teach pursed lip or diaphragmatic breathing, relaxation techniques
- Use a fan to move the air or sit the person by an open window
- Acupuncture may be helpful
- Complementary therapies.

Supportive Strategies for Constipation

- Be alert to medications that increase the risk of constipation
- Be proactive in initiating laxative therapy when opioids are initiated
- Remember that tolerance can develop, a specific laxative may become less effective over time
- When medication doses that cause constipation are titrated upward, increase anti constipation therapy
- Position so that gravity can assist with bowel movements
- Place feet on a stool when on commode or toilet
- Encourage exercise within tolerance
- Increase fluid intake if able
- Utilize dietary interventions as appropriate
- Provide privacy for defecation.

Supportive Strategies for Other Physical Symptoms

Symptom	Description	Helpful Hints
Anorexia/Loss of Appetite Anorexia is a normal occurrence at the end-of–life	• Very common • May be due to depression, unrelieved pain, mouth discomfort, difficulty swallowing, nausea, constipation, effects of chemotherapy/ radiation, changes in taste, decreased saliva production	• Small servings of favourite foods, attractively presented • Dry sherry or champagne as a stimulant • Two-handled cup or use of bendable straws • Supplements i.e. Ensure, Carnation Breakfast, milk shakes • Assist the very weak person • Check for yeast infection in the mouth Towards end of life: • Family may feel they are failing to nurture and care if they don't "encourage" the ill person to eat and drink. Explanations of the normal dying process must be given • Allowing the ill person to have what he or she wants when he or she wants it is the ideal • Frequent and thorough mouth care is necessary and required at least q1-4h
Diarrhea	• Relatively uncommon but usually due to "overflow" around a fecal impaction, viral/ bacterial infection, radiation therapy, medications (i.e. antibiotics), tumours of the colon or rectum	• Ensure that there is no fecal impaction • Dietary measures i.e. banana, yogurt, may help • Discreetly assist the person to maintain personal hygiene to avoid embarrassment as well as skin breakdown. Use barrier creams as necessary • Administer medications and treatments as ordered

Symptom	Description	Helpful Hints
Urinary frequency and/or Incontinence	• Commonly experienced by individuals with advanced malignancy • Due to bladder infections, diabetes, elevated calcium levels, pelvic tumours, radiation therapy	• Avoid embarrassing the person • Assist to bathroom every 3 – 4 hours • Use bedside commode, urinal, catheter when necessary • Protect mattress with pads • Encourage adequate fluid intake if appropriate • Use incontinence products discreetly
Urinary Retention	• May be caused by tumours obstructing the bladder, drugs (e.g. anti-depressants)	• May require catheter
Cough	• May be caused by environmental irritants (smoke, dust), dry air, lung infections/tumours • Tiring	• Sit up, prop with pillows • Try warm drink e.g. lemon and honey • Use medication as ordered
Hiccough	• Caused by spasm of the diaphragm or abdominal distension • Distressing and exhausting	• Elevate head of bed • Re-breath into paper bag • Use medication as necessary
Nausea/ Vomiting	• May be related to gastrointestinal or neurologic causes (i.e. vagal stimulation), medications (anti-inflammatory, antibiotics, iron, opioids), emotions, increased intra-cranial pressure • Often related to constipation	• Determine the cause and initiate treatment • Offer small amounts of favourite food or beverage • Ice chips, cold beverages • Calm environment • Eliminate offending odours • Medicate as necessary
Weakness	• Due to disease process, inadequate/poor nutrition, dehydration, fever, pain, chemotherapy, radiation therapy, electrolyte imbalances • Part of the dying process	• Treat cause if possible • Decrease non-essential activities • Arrange for help • Set nap times • Encourage and support but avoid nagging
Sweating	• Can be part of disease process side effect of medication	• Determine cause and treat appropriately • Check for fever • Change bedding and sleepwear as necessary • Tepid sponge/fan if fever • Medicate as necessary

Symptom	Description	Helpful Hints
Insomnia	• Usually due to unrelieved physical and/or psychological symptoms • May also be caused by prolonged bed rest or decreased diversion during late night	• Relaxing activities in evening • Decrease caffeine consumption **Physical** • Warm bath, warm drink, back rub • Hot water bottle (on feet), change position • Quiet room, soft music, shaded light **Psychological** • Reassure • Be within sight, if that helps • Talk about past or family's future • Read, watch TV, music
Mouth Pain	• May be due to local radiation therapy, chemotherapy, mouth breathing, infections (thrush), medications (e.g. antidepressants), loose-fitting dentures, poor dental hygiene	• Keep mouth clean and moist • 1 teaspoon baking soda in ¼ cup water is a good cleaning solution or mouthwash • Keep lips moist • Ice chips, favourite drink, sips of water, artificial saliva • Hard sugarless candies • Glycerine or balm for lips • Moist room air (humidifier in winter) • Treat fungal infections • Treat painful sores with analgesics
Dysphagia	• Difficulty swallowing may be related to mouth care problems, mechanical obstruction of the esophagus, tumours in the throat/chest area	• Determine cause and treat appropriately • Soft foods • Avoid fluids if choking • Thicken fluids if recommended • Treat mouth sores
Dehydration	• Related to decreased fluid intake • Common occurrence in dying process	• Support and educate the family • Have favourite fluids available if person wants. It's important not to insist that they must drink! • Give frequent mouth care
Pruritis	• Persistent itchiness may be due to excessively dry skin, jaundice, environmental and/or drug reactions	• Soothing baths/lotions • May require medication or surgical intervention

Symptom	Description	Helpful Hints
Confusion	• A complex symptom related to medication administration (e.g. tranquilizers, hypnotics, antidepressants), infections, cerebral tumours, decreased oxygen supply, cardiovascular disease, altered or unfamiliar environment	• Re-assure, point out familiar surroundings • Talk about family or other favourite topics • Maintain safety through close observation • Have someone familiar stay with the person • Consider changes in medication regime • May require diagnostic testing • Keep small light on in room at night
Skin Problems	• Due to deteriorating condition • Inactivity may lead to pressure sores	• Avoid massage over bony prominences • A mattress with low interface pressure, such as high-density foam, is recommended • For more detail and hints for skin problems refer to the RNAO Best Practice Guidelines at www.rnao.org
Bleeding	• Due to tumour infiltration of blood vessels, varices, tumour erosion, wound erosion, hemorrhage • Before evidence of bleeding, the client may become restless, confused, may yawn or pluck at bedclothes • May observe bleeding at dressing site • Blood appears like coffee grounds or grape colour when vomiting • Bowel movements appear black – tar-like	• Call professional • Reassure client and family • Keep client warm, elevate feet • Have dark or red towels on hand to absorb blood – less frightening to the person and family
Seizures	• Due to brain tumours, opioid toxicity	• Ensure safety of the person • Re-assure family • Inform professional • Medicate as necessary

Working as a Team

Seeing a person suffer with pain or other symptoms is common in hospice palliative care and can be distressing for staff, family members and friends. All members of the care team, including family and friends can observe, monitor and report. Professionals on the team have a duty to assess, share information, assist in the decision making process related to treatments, plan the care, deliver the care and confirm that the plan is acceptable to the person and that the goals are being met. Everyone on the team has a duty to advocate for the best possible symptom management.

McCaffery & Pasero, (1999) offer tips for establishing a team/collaborative approach to pain management. The tips have been adapted to relate to other symptoms as well and include:

1. Establish common goals
   - Agree on comfort/function goals for pain and /or symptom management
   - Agree that the person has the right to determine which treatments will be included in the plan
   - Develop an integrated plan of care with consideration given to every team member's input.

2. Use common language and tools
   - ESAS
   - PPS

3. Develop a common knowledge base
   - Educate professionals
   - Educate the person and family
   - Use validated assessment tools and treatment protocols.

4. Engage in routine communication
   - Respect the input of all members of the team
   - Monitor outcomes (ESAS flow sheet)
   - Maintain routine contact (e.g., daily progress report, fax, notes)
   - Use standardized report format

The whole team must work together to determine the cause of each symptom. Appropriate assessment tools should be utilized and every person on the team is responsible for reporting observations. When the symptom is related to the disease process, treat the underlying disease as appropriate.

When planning for pain management, consider the following points:

- Don't delay in treating the pain, and use multiple methods, such as:
  - modify the pathological process
  - elevate the pain threshold
  - interrupt the pain pathway
  - modify lifestyle.

- Use the WHO ladder (World Health Organization Ladder 1996)

The Analgesic Stepped Approach

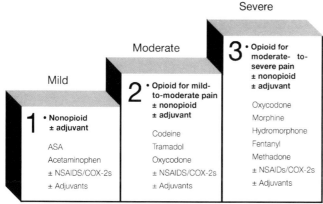

Adapted from World Health Organization 1996.

- Give medication orally whenever possible
- Chronic pain present more than 12 hours in 24 requires a constant level of analgesia so administer medications around the clock (ATC) (Mccaffery and Pasero 1999)
- Give breakthrough doses as necessary (BTD)
- Consider adjuvant therapies/treatments
- When giving analgesics to the elderly, start low and go slow
- Treat opioid side effects (constipation, nausea) aggressively
- Inform person to expect to feel somewhat sedated for a few days when opioids are begun or the dose is increased. Instruct family to notify the team if the person is difficult to rouse.

Reference List

Al-Atiyyat,N.M.H., (2009) *Cultural Diversity and Cancer Pain* Journal of Hospice and Palliative Nursing May/June 2009 Volume 11 Number 3 Pages 154 – 164

Health and Welfare Canada: *Cancer Pain: A Monograph on the Management of Cancer* (1984). Retrieved from Librach, S.L. The Pain Manual

Dudgeon, D. (2010) Dyspnea, Death Rattle and Cough. In B.R. Ferrell & N. Coyle (Eds.). *Textbook of Palliative Nursing.* New York: Oxford University Press.

Economou, D. (2010). Bowel Management: Constipation, Diarrhea, Obstruction, and Ascites. In B.R. Ferrell & N. Coyle (Eds.). *Textbook of Palliative Nursing.* New York: Oxford University Press.

Ferris, F.D., Balfour, H.M., Bowen, K., Farley, J., Hardwick, M., Lamontagne, C., Lundy, M., Syme, A., & West, P. (2002). *A model to guide hospice palliative care; Based on national principles and norms of practice.* Ottawa: Canadian Hospice Palliative Care Association.

Fink, R. & Gates, R. (2010). Pain Assessment. In B.R. Ferrell & N. Coyle (Eds.) *Textbook of Palliative Nursing.* New York: Oxford University Press.

International Association for the Study of Pain (2007). *IASP Pain Terminology.* Retrieved from www.iasp-pain.org/AM/Template.cfm?Section=Pain March 2011

Jovey, R. (2008). *Managing Pain.* Stittsville: Baker Edwards Consulting Inc.

Librach, S.L. (2007) Constipation. In Emmanuel, L. & Librach, S.L. (EDs). *Palliative Care and Core Clinical Competencies.* Philadelphia: Saunders.

McCaffery, M. & Pasero, C. (1999). *Pain: Clinical Manual for Nursing.* Toronto: Mosby.

P.I.E.C.E.S. *Putting the Pieces Together* Retrieved from www.piecescanada.com/index. php?option=com...1...

RNAO (2007) *Best Practice Guidelines for Pain Assessment and Management.* Retrieved from www.rnao. org/Page.asp?PageID=924&ContentID=720

RNAO (2011) *Complementary Therapies Nursing Interest Group.* Retrieved www.rnao-ctnig.org/ complementary-therapy.html February 2011

Schroder, C. & Dudgeon, D. (2007) Dyspnea. In Emmanuel, L. & Librach, S.L. (EDs). In *Palliative Care and Core Clinical Competencies.* Philadelphia: Saunders.

Thai, V. & Fainsinger, R. (2007) Pain. In Emmanuel, L. & Librach, S.L. (EDs). *In Palliative Care and Core Clinical Competencies.* Philadelphia: Saunders.

U.S. Department of Health and Human Services: National Institutes of Health (2007) *Constipation* NIH Publication No. 07–2754 July 2007 Retrieved from http://digestive.niddk.nih.gov/ddiseases/ pubs/constipation/ / February 2011.

ESAS-r - accessed from palliative care.org Regional Palliative Care Program Edmonton Alberta. July 2012 http://www.palliative.org/PC/ClinicalInfo/AssessmentTools/ESAS%20ToolsIdx.html

Appendix A: Pain Intensity Scales

Scale	Description	Advantages – each point represents research/studies on the scale	Disadvantages - each point represents research/studies on the scale
Visual Analogue Scale (VAS)	A vertical line of 10 cm (or 100mm) in length anchored at each end by verbal descriptors (e.g., no pain and worst possible pain). Patients are asked to make a slash mark or X on the line at the place that represents the amount of pain experienced.	Positive correlation with other self reported measures of pain intensity and observed pain behaviors. Sensitive to treatment effects and distinct from subjective components of pain. Qualities of ratio data with high number of response categories make it more sensitive to changes in pain intensity.	Scoring may e more time-consuming and involve more steps. Patients may have difficulty understanding a VAS measure. Too abstract for many adults, and may be difficult to use with elderly, non-English speaking and patients with physical disability, immobility. Or reduced visual acuity, which may limit their ability to place a mark on the line
Numeric Rating Scale (NRS)	The number that the patient gives represents his/her pain intensity from 0-10 with the understanding that 0=no pain and 10=worst pain possible.	Validity and demonstrated sensitivity to VAS. Verbal administration to patients allows those by phone or who are physically and visually disabled to quantify pain intensity. Ease in scoring high compliance, high number of response categories. Scores may be treated as interval data and are correlated with VAS.	Lack of research comparing sensitivity to treatments impacting pain intensity
Verbal Descriptor Scale (VDS)	Adjectives reflecting extremes of pain are ranked in order of severity. Each adjective is given a number which constitutes the patients pain intensity.	Short, ease of administration to patients, easily comprehended, high compliance. Easy to score and analyze data on an ordinal level. Validity is established. Sensitivity to treatments that are known to impact pain intensity.	Less reliable among illiterate patients and persons with limited English vocabulary. Patients must choose one word to describe their pain intensity even if no word accurately describes it. Variability in use of verbal descriptors is associated with affective distress. Scores on VDS are considered ordinal data; however, the distances between its descriptors are not equal but categorical.
Faces Scale (Wong Baker)	The scale consists of six cartoon-type faces. The no pain (0) face shows a widely smiling face and the most pain (10) shows a face with tears. The scale is treated as a Likert scale and was originally developed to measure children's pain intensity or amount of hurt. It has been used in adults.	Validity is supported by research reporting that persons from many cultures recognize facial expressions and identify them in similar ways. Simplicity, ease of use, and correlation with VAS makes it a valuable option in clinical settings. Short, requires little mental energy and little explanation for use.	Presence of tears on the "most" pain face may introduce a cultural bias when the scale is used by adults from cultures not sanctioning crying in response to pain.
Faces Pain Scale – Revised (FPS-R	The Faces Pain Scale Revised (FPS-R) was adapted from the FPS in order to make it compatible with a 0-10 metric scale. The FPS-R measures pain intensity consist of six oval faces ranging from a neutral face (no pain) to a grimacing sad face without tears (worst pain)	Easy to administer. Oval shaped faces without tears or wide smiles are more adult-like in appearance, possibly making the scale more acceptable adults.	Facial expressions may be difficult to discern by patients who have visual difficulties The FPS-R may measure other constructs (anger, distress. and impact on pain on functional status) than just pain intensity.
Pain Thermometer	Modified vertical verbal descriptor scale which is administered by asking the patient to point to the words that best describes his/her pain.	Increased sensitivity. Preferred for patients with moderate to severe cognitive deficits or those with difficulty with abstract thinking and verbal communication.	Allow for practice time to use this tool.

Adapted from B. Ferrell, N. Coyle – Oxford Textbook of Palliative Nursing, 3rd Edition, Oxford University Press, Inc. 2010

Chapter Five

Psychological

Psychological

- Personality, strengths, behaviour, motivation
- Depression, anxiety
- Emotions
- Fears
- Control, dignity, independence
- Conflict, guilt, stress, coping responses
- Self-image

Person and Family

- Demographics
- Culture
- Personal values, beliefs, practices and strengths
- Developmental stage, education, literacy
- Disabilities

Ferris et al., 2002

Understanding the Fundamentals

Webster's New World Medical Dictionary (2008) defines psychology as the study of the mind and mental processes, especially in relation to behaviour. Hospice palliative care examines how the mind deals with the threat of death, the process of dying, death itself, and how mental processes in such circumstances affect the behaviour of the person and family. Brescia (2007) notes that psychiatric symptoms and psychic pain (depression, anxiety and distress) are not as widely recognized as physical symptoms. People suffer needlessly, their quality of life is diminished and psychic pain adds to the distress of loved ones.

Living with a life-threatening illness is tough, demanding, and intense for loved ones as well as for the person. When provided with practical, emotional, and spiritual support through all the stages of illness, the person and family often experience privileged moments of special communication, growth, and even joy. Such moments of caring can be a shared gift; treasured by the family forever.

Emotional distress is a normal response to the diagnosis of a life-threatening illness; it can appear any time during the illness trajectory. The response may be characterised by shock, anxiety, disbelief, depression, sleep disturbances, or inability to perform activities of daily living.

Sources of distress for the person and family may include:

- Unmanaged symptoms
- Limited support
- Feelings of being a burden
- Physical limitations imposed by the illness
- Lack of control
- Lack of information
- Insensitivity by care providers
- Health care system issues
- Practical issues such as financial concerns; care of children
- Conflict in relationships

Utilization of the Edmonton Symptom Assessment System (ESAS) tool will help identify the severity of a number of components of a person's subjective psychological status such as depression, anxiety, and well-being. Synonyms for words which may be difficult for some persons to understand when scoring these particular symptoms in the ESAS tool include the following:

- Anxiety: nervousness or restlessness
- Depression: feeling blue or sad
- Well-being: overall comfort, both physical and otherwise, truthfully answering the question, "How are you?"

Anxiety

Brescia (2007) describes anxiety as a normal human response to a threat. An anxious person experiences feelings of uneasiness, uncertainty, and helplessness.

Risk Factors for Anxiety

- Fear of uncontrolled symptoms
- Altered physiologic states such as hypoxia (lack of oxygen), delirium, bleeding
- Certain medications such as steroids, antihypertensives
- Pre-existing anxiety disorder
- Some hormone secreting tumours (e.g. ACTH-secreting lung tumours) are associated with anxiety.

Assessment tools for anxiety include the Hamilton Anxiety Scale and the Beck Anxiety Scale. The tools can be downloaded from the Internet.

Depression

Depression is a well defined psychiatric illness characterized by the presence of depressed mood or loss of enjoyment, interest, or pleasure for at least two weeks, along with the presence of five specific criteria.(Brescia 2007) Four or fewer symptoms indicate a minor depression.

1. Appetite disturbance with weight gain or loss of at least 5% in 1 month.
2. Sleep disturbance
3. Motor agitation or retardation
4. Fatigue or loss of energy
5. Excessive guilt or feelings of worthlessness
6. Indecisiveness and trouble concentrating
7. Recurrent thoughts of death.

Pasacreta, Minarick and Nield-Anderson (2010) state that depression is often under recognized and under treated. Depression has the potential to decrease immune response, decrease survival time, and impair quality of life. The assessment of depression in any setting relies on the awareness of risk factors associated with depression and the ability to elicit from the person key signs, symptoms, and the history of illness. The ESAS is an excellent screening tool for depression. There are a number of assessment tools to measure depression (e.g. Hamilton Depression Rating Scale, Beck Depression Inventory, Geriatric Depression Scale, Confusion Assessment Measure(CAM). These tools can be downloaded from the internet.

Risk Factors for Depression

Brescia (2007)

- Genetic makeup

- Psychosocial stresses

- Physical disability

- Pain

- Serious medical illness

- Personal or family history of depression

- Lack of social support

- Alcoholism and/or substance abuse

- Personal history of sexual or family abuse

- Certain medications

- Poorly controlled pain

- Common in pancreatic cancer and may precede other symptoms of the disease by several months.

Dementia, Delirium and Depression

In palliative and end-of-life care, those with dementia will require special attention and screening since both depression and delirium can co-exist with dementia. It is often difficult for care providers to distinguish between dementia, delirium and depression. Dementia is defined as a gradual and progressive decline in mental processing ability that affects short term memory, communication, language, judgement, reasoning and abstract thinking. Dementia eventually affects long term memory and the ability to perform familiar tasks. There may also be changes in mood and behaviour. (Toronto Region Best Practice in LTC Initiative 2007) Delirium on the other hand is a medical emergency characterized by an acute and fluctuating onset of confusion, disturbances in attention, disorganized thinking and/or decline in level of consciousness. Delirium needs to be distinguished from a pre-existing dementia. Both delirium and dementia can be present at the same time. Delirium can be either hypoactive (unrousable, very sleepy with slowing of speech, movement and thinking), hyperactive (agitated, pacing, restless, hyperactive behaviour along with visual, auditory, tactile, gustatory or olfactory hallucinations) or mixed (combination of both manifestations). Delirium is caused by the direct physiological consequences of a general medical condition and requires prompt recognition, assessment and treatment.

Suicide

Brescia (2007) states that a clear relationship exists between depression and suicide. A sense of hopelessness is a strong risk factor and the possibility that a person with cancer will end his of her life is twice that of the general population. There is no evidence to suggest that raising the issue of suicide encourages a person to act in a self-destructive manner. Lynn, Lynch, Schuster, Wilkinson and Simon (2008) note that depression is under recognized in older adults and is often mistaken for early dementia or considered a normal part of aging. Suicide rates increase with age and depression is the key risk factor. Screening for depression is important in hospice palliative care and the ESAS is an easy tool to use for this purpose. The well-being symptom on the ESAS tool may speak to the hopelessness issue that is a risk factor for suicide in persons with cancer. Most tools used to assess depression have questions related to suicidal ideation.

Depression and anxiety may also affect other members of the family. Since the unit of care is the family, hospice palliative care providers must also monitor the mental state of the family caregivers. The caregiver's physical, emotional, and psychological exhaustion may also affect his or her ability to communicate caring, empathy, and compassion. It is important to determine how well the caregiver is coping.

Observing the Individual's Experience

The responsibility of caregivers is to identify and report the signs and symptoms that may indicate psychological distress.

The common signs and symptoms of anxiety are:

- Fear, including unrealistic fears (phobias)
- Inability to perform normal activities of daily living
- Nervousness
- Hypervigilance, excessive worry
- Restlessness, agitation
- Frequent crying spells
- Headache
- Gastrointestinal upsets
- Shortness of breath
- Palpitations
- Insomnia, trouble falling or staying asleep
- Irritability, muscle tension
- Obsessions (persistent painful ideas)
- Compulsions (repetitive ritualistic acts)
- Anorexia or over eating
- Self medicating.

Common signs of delirium are:

- Sudden onset of confusion
- Fluctuates over 24 hour period and is often worse at night
- Misperceptions and illusions
- Disturbed sleep with no set pattern
- Fluctuations in emotions (outburst, anger, fear, crying)
- May be hypoactive, hyperactive or mixed.

Common Signs and Symptoms of Depression are:

- Depressed mood; feeling sad or empty, tearful
- Decreased interest or pleasure in all or almost all activities
- Significant weight loss
- Insomnia or hypersomnia
- Psychomotor agitation or retardation
- Fatigue or loss of energy
- Feeling of worthlessness or excessive or inappropriate guilt
- Diminished ability to think or concentrate or indecisiveness
- Recurrent thoughts of death (not just fear of dying), recurrent suicidal ideation or suicide attempt (Gullatte, Kaplow, Heidrich, 2005).

Keys to determining suicide lethality include:

- Suicide plan determined
- Method chosen e.g. gun, knife, medication overdose, carbon monoxide etc.
- Intended outcome is death as opposed to rescue
- Availability of resources for treatment and support
- Ability to communicate affects the potential for success of therapy.

Severely depressed individuals must be identified quickly to ensure a safe environment and appropriate treatment. A person with an immediate, lethal and precise suicide plan needs strict safety precautions and continuous or close supervision. The motivation for suicide can be reduced by managing pain and other symptoms, referral for treatment of depression, discussion of alternative interventions to improve quality of life, referral for psychosocial spiritual care, education about the dying process and accurate facts about the options for end-of-life care and decision making. (Pasacreta et al, 2010)

Interacting with the Individual and Formal/Informal Caregivers

Attention to the principles of good communication when a person is diagnosed with a serious or life-threatening illness is paramount. The caregiver enhances communication by being fully "present" to the person and/or family. He or she needs to be sensitive to the person, making attempts to pick an appropriate time and place for conversation while acknowledging that the discussion may produce discomfort. Brescia (2007) states "The dying person takes on a special status that separates him or her from those who are seen as well and is therefore often in a state of crisis: fragile, fearful, vulnerable, wounded, dependant, time bound, and above all distressed."

Chocinov (2007) acknowledges that in our time pressured culture of modern health care the core values of kindness, humanity and respect are too often being overlooked. Dignity conserving care is a means by which to restore those values but it requires effort on the part of the healthcare provider. A person's dignity is upheld relative to the ability of the healthcare provider to see the person as is or as he or she was rather than just as the illness that has been diagnosed. When a person's dignity is not being upheld, his or her sense of value and worth are more likely to be compromised. When life no longer has meaning and purpose, the sense of being a burden to others increases and continued existence may be questioned. Chocinov uses an "A B C D" framework to help remind practitioners to not only care for people but to care about them.

Attitudes are based on perceptions that may or may not reflect the person's reality. Our perceptions frequently are based on faulty assumptions e.g. intoxication as the reason for confusion in a homeless confused person, poor quality of life in a severely disabled person, malingering in a person with chronic pain. Each healthcare practitioner needs to examine his or her attitudes and make a conscious effort to challenge and question attitudes in personal practice as well as in team practice.

Behaviours are affected by attitudes. All our actions should be predicated on kindness and respect. It doesn't take much time to perform small acts of kindness that are so meaningful to those in our care. Those with progressive life limiting illness are particularly vulnerable and simply acting in a manner that gives the person your undivided attention speaks volumes to the person about his or her worth. Asking permission of the person to perform an examination or to initiate a treatment conveys respect and dignity.

Compassion speaks to feelings that are evoked by contact with the person and how those feelings shape our approach to care. Jean Vanier the founder of L'Arche communities that focus on living with and caring for the disabled speaks of compassion as competence laced with tenderness. Compassion develops over time and can be conveyed as a gentle look or a reassuring touch that expresses recognition of the human story that accompanies illness.

Dialogue is the most important component of the framework of dignity therapy and is dependent upon the previous building blocks (ABC) being honed. Dialogue must acknowledge personhood and be intentional in portraying the recognition of the emotional impact of the illness. Getting to know the person and family, determining what is important to them and acknowledging that the effects of the illness are overwhelming at times will enhance self worth and self coherence.

Therapeutic Conversations

A therapeutic conversation takes place with a conscious intention and involves skills and knowledge on the part of caregiver. The focus of communication is on the person, not on the caregiver.

A therapeutic conversation with the person and the family related to anxiety or depression may involve the following questions:

- How are your spirits?
- What do you see for yourself in the future?
- Do you feel helpless?
- Do you feel in control?
- Do you feel like a burden?
- Are you able to fall asleep?
- Do you waken early? Do you feel refreshed when you wake up?
- Do you look forward to eating? Do you find pleasure in eating foods that you have always liked?
- Are you able to concentrate?
- Do you feel irritable or restless?
- Do you think you would be better off dead?
- Do you feel hopeless?
- Do you have any thoughts of hurting yourself?

Communication Strategies

Remember CLASS: Context, Listening, Acknowledgement of Emotion, Strategy for Management, Summary.

Outcomes of Effective Communication

When members of the team engage in therapeutic conversations with the person and family the following outcomes can be expected:

- Reduced anxiety
- Reduced isolation
- Enhanced sense of dignity
- Clarified understanding
- Informed decision making
- A relationship of trust
- Improved pain and symptom management
- Prevention of conflict

Remember: Persons with dementia require careful monitoring and any concerns about changes in behaviour or thinking expressed by family need to be taken seriously. Delirium needs to be ruled out when changes are observed and communicated.

Providing Supportive Care Strategies

Coping with personal stress in a positive manner is important for the professional caregiver and will better prepare him or her to help families and individuals cope with their stress.

There are a variety of coping mechanisms. Some people use smoking, eating, or drinking to bring a sense of immediate relief from tension; however, such strategies do not last long and the negative side effects can potentially add problems if such coping mechanisms are repeated over a long period of time. There are many strategies and therapies that promote wellbeing e.g. exercise, yoga, meditation, play, friends, journaling, art, music, drama, dance or movement therapy etc. Health practitioners can themselves endeavour to become models of effective coping. We will deal with personal and professional growth in Chapter 11.

Usually no single strategy will be effective in managing all of life's challenges. Pasacreta et al. (2010) suggest the following strategies to help to the person and family with the management of psychological distress:

1. Provide concrete, neutral information.

   - Help the person to know what to expect; fear of the unknown may be a source of anxiety
   - Encourage the person to ask questions
   - Use simple terms; avoid medical jargon
   - Repeat information as needed.

2. Prepare the person prior to a stressful event.

   - Anticipation and rehearsal of a potentially traumatic or painful experience will assist the person to maintain control and tolerate the procedure
   - Educate (within caregiver scope of practice) regarding interventions.

3. Increase opportunities for the person to maintain control.

   - Focus on what the person can control
   - Encourage decision-making regarding appointments e.g. scheduling, timing.

4. Encourage participation in care.

   - Allow the family to contribute to the care; involvement may reduce helplessness and increase sense of control. Family involvement may assist the family in recognizing and adjusting to the deterioration of the person
   - Respect cultural differences in expectations of the delivery of care
   - Respect the interest of the caregiver in participating
   - Assist family to gain expertise in expertise therapies such as relaxation and massage
   - Make certain that family caregivers have access to the numbers to call in a crisis.

5. Encourage the use of a stress diary – self-monitoring.

   - Ask the person to record circumstances, thoughts and feelings that cause stress and anxiety such as treatment-related stress, illness-related stress or unrelated stressful anxiety; this process can provide assessment information and improve working together to help the person understand thoughts and feelings.

6. Acknowledge fears
   - Listen to the person's communication of feelings
   - Create mutual support and trust
   - Reduce isolation; avoiding the anxious person or his or her fears is likely to increase vulnerability and anxiety

7. Explore near-miss events
   - A near-miss event is an upsetting experience that may overwhelm a person's ability to cope. For example, a person's own near death experience, the cardiac arrest of a person in similar circumstances, or repeated, daily, painful wound care. It is important to investigate, acknowledge fear, and realistically examine the person's situation in order to understand the reason for the anxiety.

8. Physical symptom management
   - Explore strategies that will reduce stress and allow the person to rest
   - Investigate pain as it may signal a threat (meaning of the symptom, more treatment, more fear)
   - Make certain that pain is managed, especially before a painful or frightening procedure
   - Promote self-control for managing pain, shortness of breath and fatigue
   - Use pharmacological interventions as needed
   - Recruit the support of others; refer to appropriate discipline.

9. Structure uncertainty
   - Acknowledge that this is a time of many unknowns
   - Concentrate on expected events such as meetings with caregivers, procedures, and updates.

10. Be aware of the impact of sensory deprivation
    - Be aware that signals in the environment may take on frightening meanings for the person, for example, loud noises, darkness, and marked, extended silence, may signal feelings such as abandonment or helplessness
    - Ensure that glasses and hearing aides are in place and in good working order.

11. Encourage hope
    - Recall joyous, meaningful events
    - Create a legacy; scrapbooking, videos, letter writing
    - Focus attention on others, such as the wellbeing of children or spouse
    - Focus attention on the short-term future
    - Revise goals; shifting hope from cure to comfort.

People cope successfully with the majority of their stressors, making hundreds of adjustments each day and managing most situations positively. The examples that follow are additional coping strategies that may assist the person to manage stress during life-changing situations. The ability to partake in these activities will depend upon the person's health care status.

1. Diversion
   - Spend time alone; see a movie; daydream
   - Write; paint; create something; try scrapbooking
   - Play an instrument; sing; listen to music
   - Play a game; visit with friends.

2. Family
   - Accept the good with the bad
   - Take time to be together; build family traditions; express affection
   - Share feelings.

3. Interpersonal
   - Believe in self; trust others
   - State needs and wants
   - Show feelings; share feelings
   - Accept others' boundaries; drop some involvements
   - Share problems with others
   - Ask for support from others.

4. Mental
   - Look for the humour
   - Set clear goals; hope for the best; plan for all the possibilities
   - Take charge; make decisions that take into account values and meet goals
   - Seek outside help in order to ensure choices are informed; tackle problems head-on
   - Look for some good in a bad situation
   - Focus on top priorities.

5. Physical
   - Listen to the body; recognize physical limitations
   - Breathe deeply
   - Try complementary therapies

6. Spiritual
   - Find purpose and meaning in life
   - Share beliefs with others
   - Confess; ask forgiveness; pray for others; give thanks
   - Let go of little problems; learn to live with the situation
   - Set priorities
   - Spend time and energy wisely.

Working as a Team

Team members can contribute to supporting the person and family by sharing with each other their observations, interactions, and interventions. The person / family members will determine the team members with whom they will share their deepest thoughts and concerns. It may not be the person with the knowledge and skill to respond to the issue. Permission should be sought to share the information with the team. Referral to a professional team member for further assessment and management of psychological distress may be necessary.

All too often when a person with a life-limiting illness admits to being depressed, family members and health care professionals dismiss it as a natural reaction to knowing that one's life is ending. Sadness and grief are normal reactions and usually such emotions give way to others and life goes on. When feelings of grief and sadness do not give way, health professionals need to determine if there is a clinical depression (Lynn et al 2008).

An interdisciplinary team (nurses, social worker, physician, spiritual counsellor etc) approach is essential for the optimal management of depression. (Gulatte et al 2005)

Remember every team member has a role to observe, report, and share information regarding:

- Change in behaviour (e.g. restlessness, agitation, sleeplessness, change in appetite, withdrawal)
- Change in emotional state (e.g. anger, hostility, hopelessness, despair, fearfulness, profound sadness)
- Change in cognitive status (e.g. confusion, disorientation).

The ESAS tool can identify issues in the psychological domain. Referral to other experts is important when ESAS scores for depression, anxiety and wellbeing remain high in spite of interventions by the primary team.

Reference List

Brescia, F. (2007) Depression, Anxiety, and Delirium. In L. Emmanuel and S.L. Librach (Eds), *Palliative Care Core Skills and Clinical Competencies*. Philadelphia: Saunders.

Chocinov, H. (2007) *Dignity and the essence of medicine: the A,B,C, and D of Dignity conserving care.* Retrieved from www.bmj.com/content/335/7612/184.full March 2011

Ferris, F.D., Balfour, H. M., Bowen, K., Farley, J., Hardwick, M., Lamontagne, C., Lundy, M., Syme, A., & West, P. (2002). *A model to guide hospice palliative care; based on national principles and norms of practice.* Ottawa: Canadian Hospice Palliative Care Association.

Gullatte, M., Kaplow, R., Heidrich, D.(2005) Oncology. In Kuebler, K., Dacvis, M., Moore, C. *Palliative Practices An Interdisciplinary Approach.* St. Louis: Elsevier Mosby

Lynn, J., Lynch Schuster, J., Wilkinson, A., Noyes Simon, L. (2008) *Improving Care for the End of Life A Sourcebook for health care mangers and clinicians.* New York: Oxford University Press.

Pasacreta, J., Minarik, P., & Nield-Anderson, L. (2010). *Anxiety and Depression.* In B.R. Ferrell & N. Coyle (Eds), Textbook of palliative nursing. New York: Oxford University Press.

Toronto Regional Best Practice in LTC Initiative. (2007) Recognizing Delirium, Depression and Dementia (3Ds) Retrieved from www.opadd.on.ca/Local%20Projects/documents/LocalProjects-Educ.Training-3Dscomparisonchart.pdf April 2011.

Webster's New World Medical Dictionary (2008) *Psychology.* New Jersey: Wiley Publishing Inc.

Chapter Six

Social

Person and Family

- Demographics

- Culture

- Personal values, beliefs, practices and strengths

- Developmental stage, education, literacy

- Disabilities

Social

- Cultural values, beliefs, practices

- Relationships, roles with family/friends, community

- Isolation, abandonment, reconciliation

- Safe environment

- Privacy, intimacy

- Routines, recreation, vacation

- Legal issues

- Family/caregiver protection

- Guardianship, custody issues

Ferris et al., 2002

Understanding the Fundamentals

There are many issues that fall under the social domain. We will concentrate primarily on the issues of family roles and relationships and the legal issues related to the illness journey.

The experience of facing a life-threatening illness may be overwhelming for both the person and his or her family. "It is within the psychosocial context, not the disease, that people truly live their lives."(Loscalzo, 2007) In order to assist them with the complex issues involved, caregivers need to recognize the individuality of the person and the uniqueness of the family system. Each family has unique patterns of interaction and coping and the family members have usual roles and responsibilities, formal and informal.

REMEMBER: The definition of "family" is determined by the person with the illness and includes whomever the person deems to be family. The family can include spouse, children, partner, blood relatives, neighbours, friends, and/or pets.

Family Roles and Relationships

In hospice palliative care, the person and the family are a "unit of care". The person and his or her family can be viewed as a system that functions according to many internal and external influences. Facing a life-threatening illness is not just a medical event. It is also a human experience for the person and family members as they work through the many losses that are experienced along the illness trajectory. The family members will experience changes in their roles and relationships throughout the illness; some may need to add caregiving and / or additional household duties to their usual roles. (Glass, Claxton and Rancour, 2010). The impact of a family member dying and the effect of his or her death have significant implications for the functioning of the family system. All family members can experience feelings of abandonment, anger, and frustration and need to face their own losses. Each member of the family may be at a different point in the process of coping and they may not always be able to support one another.

Gaining an understanding of the family unit is an important step to providing support.

The RNAO Best Practice Guideline, Supporting and Strengthening Families through Expected and Unexpected Life Events, advises us to remember that each family is unique and that the assessment process is a continually evolving process of data collection as family needs change. The ways in which a family will deal with progressive illness, dying and death will depend on the family's characteristics, prior experiences, developmental level and personal resources which all interact with the environment. *Appendix A* outlines questions to ask as part of a family assessment.

Cultural Beliefs, Values, and Practices

Culture refers to learned patterns of behaviours, beliefs and values shared by individuals in a particular social group. (Bowman 2007). Culture provides us with a sense of identity and belonging and gives us a framework with which to understand our experiences. Canada is a multicultural country and as such, health care providers must remember that differences in beliefs, values and traditional health care practices between the health team and the person and family have the potential to cause serious harm. The Canadian healthcare system subscribes to a western value system that holds autonomy (the right to make personal choices) and truth telling as sacred tenants. Individuals from non-western cultures may have no understanding of our approach when we come with detailed information and expect decisions to be made by the capable person him or herself. They may find the approach totally foreign and conflict can arise.

In health care, specifically hospice palliative care, a person's culture may have effects on (College of Nurses of Ontario, 2004):

- Perception of health, illness
- Meaning and role of suffering
- View of hospitals, health care providers, healers
- Rituals and customs
- Expressions of loss, grief (e.g. the words "death" and "dying" may not be accepted)
- Boundaries regarding privacy, age, gender, and relationships
- Effectiveness and values of therapies
- Time-keeping beliefs
- Family and social relationships (roles, hierarchies)
- Decision-making, consent to treatment (e.g. some families have decisions made by one person, others may use a more collaborative approach)
- Independence/self-care vs. interdependence
- Communication norms (eye contact, asking questions, who speaks).

Caregivers must avoid grouping or stereotyping people from a particular race, ethnicity, or professional group. Members of the same ethnic group or profession may have totally different values and beliefs. It is most important to ask rather than assume. Though individuals from various ethnic groups make up our Canadian population and have different perceptions about health care, we are bound by specific laws that impact how we go about providing health care.

Legal Concepts

The following definitions are derived from the Heath Care Consent Act in Ontario (2006)

Treatment

Treatment is defined as anything that is done for a therapeutic, preventative, palliative, diagnostic, cosmetic, or other health-related purpose, including a course of treatment or a plan of treatment All treatments require informed consent.

Informed Consent

A consent to treatment is informed if, before giving it, the person received information about:

1. the nature of the treatment

2. the expected benefits of the treatment

3. the material risks of the treatment

4. the material side effects of the treatment

5. alternative courses of action

6. the likely consequences of not having the treatment

The person must also have received responses to his or her requests for additional information.

Consent to treatment is always given by the capable person. In order for consent to be valid, it must relate to the treatment. It must be informed. It must be given voluntarily and not be obtained through misrepresentation or fraud. By following the letter of the law and insisting on providing information necessary to make an informed consent to individuals who do not want all the details, we would cause harm. Therefore, for cultural or other reasons, it is justifiable for the health care professional to provide all the information necessary to make an informed decision to another appropriate person. That person then makes the decision related to treatment. The health professional then must go to the person from whom consent was required and explain that the conversation resulted in a decision to have, withhold or withdraw a specific treatment. The person would then be asked to confirm his or her consent to the plan.

Capacity

According to the Health Care Consent Act, a person has capacity to consent if that person is capable of:

- Understanding the information that is relevant to making a decision about the treatment
- Appreciating the reasonably foreseeable consequences of a decision or a lack of decision.

A person who is capable of providing consent is also capable of withdrawing consent to the treatment. The person may be capable of consenting to some treatments and not others depending on the complexity of the decision. A person may lose capacity and regain capacity.

Substitute Decision Maker (SDM)

Prior to any treatment being initiated, consent is required. If the person is capable, then he or she makes the decision. If the person is incapable, then the health care provider refers the decision making to the substitute decision maker.

The substitute decision maker is determined according to a hierarchy set out in the Health Care Consent Act.

1. The guardian of the person if the guardian has authority to give or refuse consent
2. The Attorney for Personal Care if the Power of Attorney (the document) confers authority to give or refuse consent
3. A representative of the consent and capacity board
4. The incapable person's spouse or partner
5. A child or parent or children's aid society. All children have equal ranking. If children disagree with one another about a decision, the Consent and Capacity Board representative will make the decision in their stead.
6. A parent of a child with right of access
7. A brother or sister
8. Any other relative
9. Public guardian and trustee.

Meaning of Spouse:

Two persons are spouses if:

- They are married to each other; or
- They are living in a conjugal relationship outside of marriage and,
  - have cohabited for at least one year
  - are together the parents of a child, or
  - have together entered into a cohabitation agreement under the Family Law Act

Two persons are not spouses if they are living separate and apart as a result of a breakdown of their relationship.

Meaning of Partner:

A partner is either of two persons who have lived together for a least a year and have a close personal relationship that is of primary importance in both persons' lives.

Meaning of Relative:

Two persons are relatives if they are related by blood, marriage or adoption.

The SDM may give or refuse consent only if he or she is:

- Capable with respect to the treatment
- Is at least 16 years old or is the incapable person's parent
- Is not prohibited by court order or separation agreement from access or giving or refusing consent
- Is available (a person is available if it is possible, within a time that is reasonable for the circumstances to communicate with the person and obtain consent or refusal)
- Is willing to assume the responsibility

Principles for Giving or Refusing Consent

If the SDM knows of a wish applicable to the circumstances that the incapable person expressed while capable and after reaching the age of 16, the SDM shall give or refuse consent based on the known wishes. If the SDM does not know of a wish applicable to the circumstance or it is impossible to comply with the wish, the SDM shall act in the person's best interest.

Best Interests

In deciding what the incapable person's best interests are, the SDM shall take into consideration:

- The person's values and beliefs
- Whether the treatment is likely to:
  - Improve the person's condition or well-being
  - Prevent the person's condition from deteriorating
  - Reduce the extent or rate at which deterioration is likely
- Whether the condition is likely to improve remain the same or deteriorate without the treatment
- Whether the benefit of the treatment outweighs the risk of harm
- Whether a less restrictive or less intrusive treatment would be just a beneficial as the one proposed

The SDM is entitled to receive the same information required for an informed consent as would be given to the capable person.

Confidentiality

On November 1, 2004, the (PHIPA) came into force. The purpose of PHIPA is to provide consistent and comprehensive rules governing the collection, use, retention, disclosure and disposal of personal health information in the custody and control of health information custodians. The Privacy Act (2006) "extends the present law in Canada that protects the privacy of an individual and provides the individual with a right of access to personal information about themselves".

Confidentiality refers to the person's right to expect that what happens or is disclosed between him or her and health care providers will not be discussed with anyone else unless permission to do so has been given. Sometimes sensitive information that a care provider has acquired may be important to the other members of the care team in order to help them better understand or care for the person. Information shared to facilitate future care is usually thought of as within the boundaries of confidentiality. If a formal caregiver has been given sensitive information, it is important to let the person know why it is important to share the information and ask the person for permission to share the information. Maintaining confidentiality can be challenging for a specific care provider on the team when personal information disclosed may benefit the provision of care by some members of the team but not necessarily all members. In smaller communities, where everyone knows everyone, confidentiality can be very challenging. For instance, when a health care provider is asked about a person's situation by a neighbour, friend or even a family member of the ill person, the care provider must not be rude but must be clear about the responsibility to maintain confidentiality. By politely acknowledging the rules of confidentiality, the care provider is demonstrating that he or she is a professional and can be trusted. Various professional colleges have ethical principles and standards around privacy and confidentiality and other members of the team such as PSWs and volunteers are required to sign agreements related to confidentiality as part of their employment or association with a hospice or other organization.

Legal Documents

The following documents are frequently referred to in the process of providing hospice palliative care and are specifically related to Ontario legislation. There are variances in legislation between different provinces, states and countries.

A **Power of Attorney for Personal Care** (POAPC) is a document in which a person names an Attorney for Personal Care. The attorney named in the document takes on the responsibilities of the substitute decision maker only when the person becomes incapable of providing consent. Personal care includes health care, nutrition, shelter, clothing, hygiene, and safety. The person(s) named in the document becomes the substitute decision maker (SDM) for personal care decisions when the person becomes incapable. Wishes about future health and personal care can be documented on the form. The POAPC document must be signed and dated and witnessed by two people. Forms are available free of charge from the office of the Public Guardian and Trustee.

An **Advance Directive** or **Living Will** is a document in which wishes about future care are expressed. This document can help the substitute decision maker make decisions based on the person's wishes when that person cannot make decisions for himself or herself. Wishes need not be documented but can be provided verbally, recorded or through any means of communication. Later wishes prevail. It is important that those who will have to make decisions in the event of incapacity be apprised of the person's wishes, goals, and beliefs.

Living wills and advance directives do **NOT** speak to the health care team but are directives given to the substitute decision maker. The danger in providing the health care provider with advance directives, a living will or other levels of care documents is that the information may be used by the physician in determining what treatment options to offer or by the nurse in determining whether or not to report symptoms to the physician. This is not a legitimate use of such documents. The health care provider who knows of the advance care directives or goals and values of the person can assist in the decision making process by sensitively referring to the wishes and directives when a decision has to be made either by a capable person or the SDM about treatment for a current condition.

Each new issue that arises along the illness trajectory requires discussion and consent to a plan of treatment related to the current health care situation. A capable person or the SDM in cases of incapacity can consent to a plan of treatment for end-of-life care in which specific treatments are withheld or withdrawn. This is only appropriate if the particular disease process will lead to the need for the treatment being discussed. Examples might be: a person with ALS has indicated a wish never to have a feeding tube inserted. He or she may be provided with all the information necessary in order to make an informed decision because the disease trajectory for ALS includes loss of the ability to swallow. He or she may consent to a plan of treatment to withhold the feeding tube. However when the actual time comes when a feeding tube is indicated, the person should again be given the option to change his or her mind. However, if the person is incapable, the former plan of treatment would need to be upheld by the team unless the SDM could provide evidence that the person had changed his or her mind and had withdrawn consent.

A **Continuing Power of Attorney for Property** is a legal document in which a capable person authorizes an individual or individuals to make financial decisions on his or her behalf. The Attorney for Property can make decisions related to finances, home, and possessions. The POAP (document) comes into effect when signed unless otherwise stated and gives authority for the person named to continue to act even when the person becomes incapable. The document must name one or more persons, be signed and dated by the capable person, and be signed by two witnesses who saw the person sign the document.

Advance Care Planning (ACP)

ACP is a process of planning for a time when a person no longer has the mental capacity to make decisions about aspects of his or her care or treatment. ACP may involve planning for end-of-life care as well as care during an extended period of time of incapacity and should involve the discussion of diagnosis, prognosis, expected course of illness, possible treatment alternatives and risks/benefits of each treatment, all of which should be placed in the context of the person's goals, expectations, fears, values, and beliefs.

Steps involved in Advance Care Planning include:

1. Consideration of your values, goals, beliefs

2. Consultation with people you trust who can give you guidance e.g. your doctor, your lawyer, your faith leader

3. Consideration of whom you could trust to make the decisions you would want them to make if you were capable

4. Communication of your goals, values and wishes about future care with your family and friends as well as your health care providers

5. Appointing a substitute decision maker in a Power of Attorney for Personal Care if you want to name a specific person or person to make decisions if you become incapable

6. Ensuring that your SDM and family are aware of your goals, wishes, and values.

Another legal issue that sometimes arises in the care of those with progressive life-limiting illness are the issues of physician assisted suicide and euthanasia. Both physician assisted suicide and euthanasia are criminal offences in Canada.

Physician assisted suicide is described by Dr. Nuala Kenny (2007) as an act which involves a physician providing the means for a person to end life either by prescribing a lethal dose of medication or furnishing information to enable the person to perform the act that causes death. It is the person who completes the act which ends the life. She goes on to explain that euthanasia involves the health care provider performing an intervention, usually a lethal injection that will end the person's life. Euthanasia can be categorized as voluntary, involuntary or non-voluntary.

• Voluntary euthanasia is requested by the person.

• Involuntary euthanasia is performed despite the objection of the person.

• Non-voluntary euthanasia occurs when the person's decision has not been sought e.g. when those to be euthanized lack capacity.

Dr. Kenny contends that it is the phenomenal advances in medical science and technology of the 20th century that have caused the debate. The same technologies that can save life can prolong dying. "The technological imperative, with its bias for interventions, dominates the thinking of the public and health professionals alike."(Kenny 2007) Meier (2010) contends that debates about euthanasia date back to at 400 B.C. with the Hippocratic Oath which states, "I will give no deadly medicine to anyone if asked, nor suggest any such counsel." In recent times, public anxiety about end-of-life care, fear of loss of control once one is in the medical care system, and rising demands for self-determination have led to a resurgence of the debate. A number of Canadians, alarmed about suffering associated with dying, are beginning to consider euthanasia and assisted suicide as a means of ending suffering by deliberately causing death. Canadian law currently prohibits both physician assisted suicide and euthanasia but the case for euthanasia and physician assisted suicide has been brought before the senate and the legislature in recent years. Though there are advocates of changing the law, the Canadian Hospice Palliative Care Association does not support these approaches. Hospice palliative care, with the focus on relieving suffering, has the goal of improving quality of life, so that a person does not view ending his or her life as the best or only option.

Hospice palliative care supporters restrict the definition of euthanasia to situations in which there is intent to end life. Managing pain and other symptoms with doses of medications that could possibly hasten the death is NOT euthanasia or assisted suicide. The medication is given for the sole purpose of managing the distress caused by the symptom. The unintended effect of the medication may lead to a hastened death. This is based on the ethical principle known as the principle of the double effect.

Hospice palliative care never intentionally ends life but supports the following compassionate care interventions which are focused on providing comfort and maintaining dignity, knowing that death will occur naturally:

- Allowing refusal/withdrawal of treatment by a competent individual/substitute decision-maker

- Allowing refusal/withdrawal of treatment through an advanced directive to a substitute decision maker

- Allowing the withholding or withdrawing of treatment deemed futile or of no benefit or if it is causing harm

- Allowing appropriate pain and symptom management (including palliative sedation when other methods of treatment fail) to be provided without legal liability.

Observing the Individual's Experience

Observation of the person's and family's physical and emotional environment will help to inform the formal caregivers about such things as relationship issues, role difficulties, cultural beliefs and practices. It is important to be aware of:

- Items suggesting the importance of cultural practices

- Family photos, greeting cards from family, friends

- Regular or frequent visitors/no visitors

- Family members providing care – comfortable/reluctant/avoiding

- Interactions – comfortable/tense

- Strained/warm relationships

- Exhausted/managing caregivers

- Family gatherings

- Interactions between parents and children

- Chaotic, strained/peaceful atmosphere.

One of the important observations team members are called upon to note is the coping strategies of various members of the family. Our task is to observe without prejudice and not make judgements about coping strategies. Coping strategies are neither right nor wrong; good nor bad. Remember the way in which the person and other members of the family approach life and death is a choice. As skilled care givers we can be alert for opportunities that invite deeper investigation and more realistic communication.

Interacting with the Individual and Formal/Informal Caregivers

Persons and family members living with chronic progressive illness will often voice concerns about the future and share information about emotional and family problems to other members of the interdisciplinary team rather than to the physician. They may not want to burden the doctor or nurse with concerns that they consider unrelated to the disease process itself. The roles of various members of the team are delineated by the person and family and they will act accordingly. Though all members of the team need to observe and report expressed concerns and symptoms, the volunteer or the PSW may be the one who first becomes aware of issues in the social domain. Referral to social work is important. The social worker on the team is generally the team member with the greatest knowledge and skill to talk to the person about emotions, family problems, and psychosocial concerns.

In terms of issues related to the legal aspects of care at the end of life, it is important for the topics of goals, values, beliefs, substitute decision making, advance directives to be discussed early in the illness trajectory and as the illness progresses in order to avoid conflict between family members or between family and the health care team. The health care team will need to ascertain, who the substitute decision maker is in the event that the person becomes incapable. During a crisis is not the time to be discerning who the legal substitute decision maker is or what the goals and values of the person are.

Starks, Vig and Pearlman (2007) offer the following advice around advance care planning.

Who should initiate the conversation?

Any clinician can initiate the conversation. Different expertise and points of entry are brought to the case by physicians, case managers, nurses and social workers. The medical facts and available treatment options are best discussed by the physician who knows the person's condition and the probable trajectories of the illness as well as the range of options and outcomes of various treatments. Nurses are often the ones who explore the psychosocial aspects and elicit information about values and goals. They can offer answers to questions, clarify misunderstandings, explain details of medical treatments and revisit any topics addressed in previous discussions. Social workers may introduce the topic of advance care planning and help the person complete legal documents. They are also adept at leading family conferences and have the skills to negotiate differences of opinion among family members and gain consensus about changing goals of care.

What communication strategies are best?

Good communication skills are vital to the process. Particularly necessary in this discussion are being able to listen without interruptions, being open to questions, being sensitive to when persons chose to engage or not to engage, using plain and honest language, ensuring that the person and family understand what is being said and appearing comfortable when talking about death and dying.

How should the topics be introduced?

Normalizing the topic and being comfortable with the subject puts the person at ease. It is important to explain why the topic is being introduced.

Possible Scripts

Routine Visit with no Recent Changes in Health Status

You seem to be doing well right now and I have no reason to believe that things will change in the next while, but I do like to talk to all my patients about their preferences for care in case they get very sick. I think it is best to talk about these things when you are feeling well and before we need to react in a crisis. That gives both of us time to talk about what matters to you. I would like to give you the kind of care that you want in the future. Would it be okay to talk about this today?

Episode of Acute Illness or Hospitalization

It's vital that we work together when you are so sick. It may be hard to think about these things right now but it is really important that I understand your goals. Would it be okay if we talk about this right now?

Follow-up Visit after Illness Exacerbation

You were pretty sick last time I saw you. Are you feeling better now? At times like this I like to talk about goals of care to make sure that I'm up to date with what you would want in case you have another episode like that and others have to make decisions for you. Would it be okay to talk about this now?

Specific Questions to elicit Preferences and Goals of Care

- Have you completed a Power of Attorney for Personal Care? If yes: Who have you named as your attorney for personal care? If no: Who would you like to make decisions for you if you are incapable? If the person stated is the SMD according to the hierarchy then the person doesn't need to formally appoint him or her in a legal document.

- What is your understanding of your current condition?

- What are your hopes about your illness?

- What are your fears about how the illness will affect you in the future?

- Are there any situations in which you would rather die than be kept alive with life sustaining treatments? Why do you feel that way?

- Are there any treatments that you would not want under any circumstances? Why?

- When hearing about the illness or deaths of others, have you ever said to yourself, "I sure wouldn't want to live like that"? What made you say that?

- What are your past experiences of caring for someone who was very sick? What did you learn from those experiences that inform how you would like to be cared for?

- Who would you count on for support? Are there family, friends, religious or spiritual advisors that you would want to be involved in your care?

- What are your goals?

- Are there specific beliefs or values that might affect your decisions about any treatments?

- Have you discussed these things with your spouse, family, or friends? Should we arrange a time to talk to your family about your wishes and goals in the event that you have a sudden change in your condition just so we are all on the same page?

It is important to inform the person that consent is required for treatments before they are initiated and the person if capable can always change his or her mind. If the person is incapable the SDM is required to follow the last known wishes when consenting to treatment.

What if the person or family is reluctant to talk about these issues?

Possible reasons

- Cultural issues may discourage talking about bad news
- The coping mechanism used in the situation is to avoid thinking about dying or death
- Unwillingness to discuss because talking about future distracts from the present
- No point in speculating about the future when it cannot be controlled.

Exploration of preferences

- Focus on the role of the substitute decision maker and how that person in keeping with the law needs to know the wishes
- Talk to the person about hoping for the best but planning for possibilities
- Use "ask-tell-ask" and "tell me more" strategies to illicit hopes and fears.

If the person does not wish to engage in discussions, it is reasonable to inform the person that when consent to treatments are required in the future, the information will be provided to the capable person or in cases of incapacity, to the SDM. If the SDM does not know the person's wishes, he or she will be required to make the decisions based on the person's best interests at the time. It is also reasonable to point out to the person that knowledge of wishes is very helpful for the SDM since he or she knows what decision the person would make in various situations. Having a clear understanding eases the burden of responsibility.

Supportive Care Strategies

Establishing what the person and family knows and understands about the disease and its prognosis provides clues as to how each person is coping. When family members collude in withholding the truth from the person, it is generally out of love and because they cannot face the truth. Approaching collusion from this perspective makes it possible to respect the family member's reasons and work positively with them. (McGuire & Weiner 2009) The first step is to acknowledge the collusion. Ask: "Why do you think that... ought not to know that he is dying?" Check out if there are emotional costs as a result of the collusion. Ask: "Can I ask what effect this has been having on you personally? If there is evidence of emotional strain or an effect on the relationship, ask if the person would like you to suggest how the situation could be handled. Indicate that you would like to have a chat with the person about his or her understanding of what is happening and ask if the family member would like to be present. Emphasize that you have no intention of telling the person and if necessary enter into a contract to that effect but also indicate that you will not lie if directly asked. Very often the person's perception is that of a deteriorating condition but he or she wants to protect the family by not talking about it. Breaking collusion is difficult but it can lead to finishing business, strengthening relationships and a more positive grief experience for the family following the death.

Denial is used as a defence mechanism when the truth is too painful to bear and as such, it need not be challenged unless it is causing serious problems for the person or member(s) of the family. In challenging denial, be gentle but explore any awareness. Ask the person to relate what has happened since the illness was first discovered and explore how it felt at each key point as well as the perceptions of what was wrong. Phrases such as "pretty sure" or "I think" can be repeated back to the person for further clarification. If any ambivalence is uncovered, it is appropriate to acknowledge that by indicating that it appears that part of the person prefers to believe the situation is not serious but another part considers that things are getting worse. Ask how the person would like you to relate to him or her. It is appropriate to challenge the incongruence between perceptions and experiences. If that doesn't work look for a window of opportunity. If the person seems discouraged, ask if there is ever a moment when he or she feels that the situation may not be as simple as wished. Assisting the person to shift from denial to reality can be very satisfying for the team member but it is important to determine whose needs are being met.

In terms of addressing legal issues, decision making capacity is an aspect of care in which all members of the team can participate. Those who spend considerable time with the person may be the first to observe signs of incapacity. Language barriers also need to be identified and using family members to translate should be avoided. Ensure that translators are aware that they should accurately translate what has been said and not change the words in an attempt to soften the message.

Other supportive strategies include:

- Attempting to anticipate questions the family or person may ask and being emotionally prepared to discuss social issues / concerns
- Frequently asking the person and family to identify any concerns, unaddressed issues and priorities
- Bringing any questions or misunderstanding about the illness or its treatment to the team
- Making referrals to appropriate team members to address social issues
- If the person is in a facility e.g. hospital, long term care home, enhance the environment to support quality of life and be hospitable to family and friends.

Working as a Team

Communicating the PPS among team members will help to inform the team of declining functional status which may indicate impending death. Generally, if PPS scores decline over months or weeks, the person has months or weeks to live. If the PPS changes over days, the person may have only days to live.

Each member of the team has an important part to play in:

- alerting the team to problems that the person or family are not able or willing to share with professionals
- advocating for quality of life by communicating all symptoms, side effects, observations and concerns with the rest of the health care team in a timely manner
- educating the person and family in order to debunk myths and enable them make decisions based on research and best practice guidelines as well as personal values and goals

There are many decisions to make once a person is told he or she has a terminal illness. Often people feel overwhelmed and alone in making those decisions, wondering how to involve those they care about, fearful of asking for help from others or participating in the decision-making process.

One way to pursue this decision-making process is to have a family meeting / conference. The person, a trusted family member or friend, or a health care professional will usually initiate a family conference. Any member of the team can be invited to participate in the meeting, including the social worker or spiritual advisor.

A family meeting or conference can be arranged:

- after the diagnosis is made
- any time an issue causes significant challenges; the conference can be initiated by health care providers or by the person and/or family
- when an important intervention or change of treatment is considered
- when the person has had a significant deterioration that may suggest the appropriateness of a change in focus or direction of the medical management.

Reference List

Bowman, K. (2007) Understanding and Respecting Cultural Differences. In Emmanuel, E. And Librach, S.L. *Palliative Care Core Skills and Competencies.* Philadelphia: Saunders Elsevier

College of Nurses of Ontario. (2004). *Practice guidelines: Culturally Sensitive Care.* Toronto:

College of Nurses of Ontario.

Ferris, F.D., Balfour, H.M., Bowen, K., Farley, J., Hardwick, M., Lamontagne, C., Lundy, M., Syme, A., & West, P. (2002). *A model to guide hospice palliative care; Based on national principles and norms of practice.* Ottawa: Canadian Hospice Palliative Care Association.

Glass, E., Cluxton, D., Rancour, P. (2010). Principles of patient and family assessment. In B.R. Ferrell & N. Coyle (Eds.). *Textbook of palliative nursing.* New York: Oxford University Press.

Government of Canada (2006). Privacy Act. Retrieved July, 2006 from http://laws.justice.gc.ca/en/p-21/text.html.

Government of Ontario (1996) Health Care Consent Act. (amended 1998, 2000, 2002, 2004, 2006) Retrieved from www.e-laws.gov.on.ca/html/.../elaws_statutes_96h02_e.htm - Cached

Government of Ontario (1992) Substitute Decisions Act. Retrieved from www.e-laws.gov.on.ca/html/.../elaws_statutes_92s30_e.htm - Cached - Similar

Kenny, N., (2007) Responding to Requests for Euthanasia and Assisted Suicide. In Emmanuel, E. And Librach, S.L. *Palliative Care Core Skills and Competencies.* Philadelphia: Saunders Elsevier

Loscalzo, M. (2007) *Social Workers: The Connective Tissue of the Health Care System.* In Emmanuel, E. And Librach, S.L. *Palliative Care Core Skills and Competencies.* Philadelphia: Saunders Elsevier

Maguire, P. & Weiner, J. (2009) Communication with Terminally Ill Patients and their Families. In Chocinov, H. & Brietbart, W. (Eds) *Handbook of Psychiatry in Palliative Medicine.* New York: Oxford University Press.

RNAO Best Practice Guideline, *Supporting and Strengthening Families through Expected and Unexpected Life Events.* Retrieved from http://www.rnao.org/Storage/15/945_BPG_Family_supplement.pdf

Starks, H., Vig, E., & Pearlman, R. (2007) *Advance Care Planning.* In Emmanuel, E. & Librach, S.L. Palliative Care Core Skills and Competencies. Philadelphia: Saunders Elsevier

Appendix A

Sample Questions for Key Areas of Family Assessment: RNAO Best Practice Guideline Supporting and Strengthening Families

Identifying data (Names, ages, addresses - Who is the primary person to contact? Does the family have any transportation difficulties?)

Composition (Family Unit - Could you tell me who is in the family? Is there anyone else who is not related that you think of as family? How close is the family?)

Culture/ethnicity (Knowledge and customs of family - Could you tell me about the family's cultural background? Does ethnicity influence the family's health beliefs? Are there any ethnic customs the family gains strength from or may need assistance with?)

Spiritual identification (Characteristic values of a person which may or may not be a religious affiliation - Are your spiritual beliefs a resource for family members? Is there anyone that can be contacted to assist the family with their spiritual needs?)

Economic status (Income of family - Who is (are) the breadwinner(s) in the family? Is the family able to meet current and future needs? What type of work?)

Lifestyle and health behaviours (Nutrition, drugs and alcohol, smoking, activity and rest)

Developmental stage (Family's present developmental stage and developmental stage history [e.g. births, retirement, aging parents, deaths], extent to which the family is fulfilling the developmental tasks appropriate for their developmental stage)

Power and role structures (Who makes what decisions? Are family members satisfied with how decisions are made and who makes them? What positions and roles do each of the family members fulfill? Is there any role conflict? How are family tasks divided up?)

Communication (Family's ability to interact with one another - Are family members able to communicate openly with one another? Is conflict openly expressed and discussed? Do family members respect one another?)

Home characteristics (Type of characteristics of the home - Can you describe your home? Do you own or rent? Do you consider your home adequate for your needs?)

Community characteristics (Describe your neighbourhood/community, e.g. rural or urban, schools, recreation, access to health care, crime rate, environmental hazards, etc.?)

Health patterns (Family's health beliefs, values and behaviours - How does the family assess their present health status? What present health problem(s) does the family identify?)

Values (Family's fundamental ideas, opinions, and assumptions - What values/beliefs does the family have that have assisted them in adapting successfully or unsuccessfully?)

Coping mechanisms (Ability to adapt to stress and maintain emotional well-being and stability of its members - How has the family coped with past crises? What helped the most and the least? What strengths does the family have to assist in coping? Do family members differ in their ways of coping?)

Problem solving (Family's ability to organize a stressor into manageable components and to identify courses of action to solve it effectively - How has the family resolved problems in the past? What resources have they used?)

Family Resources and Capabilities (Resources the family use to assist adapting to the stressor - What intra, inter and extrafamilial resources are the family using and require information on?)

Family appraisal of the stressor (What is the family's estimate of the strength and duration of the stressor?)

Major concerns (What are the family's major concerns?)

Chapter Seven

Domain: Spiritual

Person and Family

- Demographics
- Culture
- Personal values, beliefs, practices and strengths
- Developmental stage, education, literacy
- Disabilities

Spiritual

- Meaning, value
- Existential, transcendental
- Values, beliefs, practices, affiliations
- Spiritual advisors, rites, rituals
- Symbols, icons

Ferris et al., 2002

Understanding the Fundamentals

Hospice Palliative Care supports the tenant that personal growth along the illness journey is possible. Such growth occurs in spite of or perhaps even because of suffering (Hallenbeck, 2003). The diagnosis of a life-threatening illness, accompanied by loss, separation, suffering, and loneliness can lead to spiritual distress. That same distress may be the springboard to growth in spirit that caregivers witness in many persons who are living with dying.

Dying for most people involves spiritual work. The diagnosis of a life-threatening illness can raise questions about beliefs and values, the meaning of suffering, mortality, life after death and relationships. It is the spiritual part of us that seeks answers to such questions and longs for meaning and purpose in our lives.

A person's spiritual nature challenges him or her to explore questions such as:

- Who am I?
- Do I have meaning?
- What is my role and purpose in this world?
- Is there a higher power?
- What happens after death?
- Why is this happening to me?

Death and dying have been reflected upon since the advent of written history. People die today with the same concerns, struggles and fears that millennia ago were recorded in various Books of the Dead. The books (Gnostic, Tibetan, Egyptian and Medieval Monastic) all reflect universal themes that transcend culture and spirituality (Groves and Klauser 2005). In the Celtic tradition, the wisdom related to the care of the dying was passed on orally. Celts saw a parallel between the birth and the death processes and employed anamcara (a soul friend) or midwife who supported both processes. In hospice palliative care, there is a growing interest in applying the wisdom of the ancestors to address the unique emotional and spiritual distress of those who are living with dying. An anamcara according to the Celtic tradition acts as a soul friend who is a spiritual companion who honours the uniqueness of the dying person's spiritual journey. Utilizing the wisdom of the ages, the soul friend offers opportunities for healing and hope at the end of life.

In the American Book of the Dying, Lessons in Healing Spiritual Pain, Groves and Klauser (2005) note that all books of the dead, regardless of culture, time and place indicate that spiritual pain is related to one of the following.

- Meaning
- Forgiveness
- Relatedness
- Hopelessness.

Meaning pain is related to the question: Who am I? Often the same spiritual pain that creates a crisis of meaning can also lead to a path out of the crisis.

Forgiveness pain is the most common spiritual pain (Groves et al. 2005). Healers of every spiritual tradition indicate that we are forgiven to the extent that we can release others. Often, the most challenging one to forgive at the end of life is oneself.

Relatedness pain refers to the suffering experienced by having to leave everything known behind. Relatedness does not refer only to personal relationships but also to relationships with possessions, roles and identities. Resisting the reality of the natural balance between darkness and light, life and death, leads to spiritual pain. By leaning into the pain rather than resisting, growth and healing is made possible (Groves & Klauser 2005). Many who have worked in hospice palliative care over the years have had "teachers" who say they would never exchange the experience of living with a progressive life limiting illness with the life they had before the diagnosis.

Hopelessness pain refers to the loss of all reason for living. Hope comes from the ability to imagine what could be life-giving. When such a desire is sustained by an expectation of fulfillment, hope results. For those living with progressive illness, there comes a time when there is a realization that functionally this is as good as it's going to get. Hopelessness may result or the person may shift priorities and give more attention to inner awareness. Dying ultimately involves recognition that the old familiar life is no longer sustainable (Groves et al 2005). Yielding enables growth and healing.

Religion and spirituality are examples of how we attempt to make sense of the world and ourselves. There are many definitions of spirituality and religion. *A Model to Guide Hospice Palliative Care* (Ferris et al., 2002) defines spirituality as:

- The way in which a person makes meaning and organizes his or her sense of self around a personal set of beliefs, values, and relationships, sometimes understood in terms of transcendence or inspiration. Involvement in a community of faith and practice may or may not be a part of an individual's spirituality.

Religion is defined by Wright (2005) as:

- The affiliation or membership in a particular faith community that shares a set of beliefs, rituals, morals, and sometimes a health code, centered on a defined higher power or transcendent power, most frequently referred to as God. An example of a health care code would be the withholding of blood transfusion in the Jehovah Witness faith.

Baird (2010) notes there is considerable discussion related to what constitutes good spiritual care and to date there are no universally agreed upon terms. The definitions she utilizes in an attempt to demystify spiritual care follow.

- Spirituality: our relationship with ourselves, others, nature and the transcendent

- Religion: an organization that has a set of rites, rules, practices, values, and beliefs that prescribe how individuals should live their lives and respond to God

- Spiritual care: allowing our humanity to touch another's humanity by providing presence, deep listening and compassion

- Compassion: the ability to be empathically present to another while he or she is suffering and is trying to find meaning

- Existential: relating to human existence and experience.

A person who is deeply spiritual may not subscribe to a particular religion. Conversely, simply acknowledging affiliation with a particular religion does not necessarily mean that the person is spiritually inclined. Some individuals may deny being spiritual and reject organized religion but virtually everyone has some sort of understanding of how the universe functions (Hallenbeck, 2003).

Finding meaning, forgiveness, relatedness and hope in illness is a unique journey for each person.

Observing the Individual's Experience

Being mindful of identifying issues in the spiritual domain is important for every caregiver regardless of his or her role. A friend, a volunteer, a personal support worker or someone cleaning the room may be the one to whom the person bares his or her soul. The choice of whether to recognize and nourish the spiritual part of our nature is a personal choice, not the choice of health care providers or family.

A rising score in well-being on the ESAS may point to spiritual distress. Other indicators of spiritual distress may include:

A sense of abandonment
- "My friends don't visit anymore."
- "My wife won't let me talk about dying!"
- "Why isn't God answering my prayers?"

Anger
- "God shouldn't allow this to happen!"
- "I hate myself for not having stopped smoking!"

Remorse
- "I wish I had spent more time with my kids!"
- "I wish I had gone to church more often."

Fear of dying
- "I'm scared."
- "I'm afraid to go to sleep."

Difficulty accepting love
- "I don't deserve this special treatment."

Discouragement
- "Why do I have to suffer like this?"
- "What's the use?"

Hopelessness
- "I wish it would all end!"
- "Why don't you just give me something to end it all?"

Withdrawal and isolation
- "Leave me alone!"
- "Leave the blinds closed!"

Doubt
- "I wonder if there really is a God?"

There are a number of spiritual assessment tools that can be used if the caregiver suspects spiritual pain is an issue that needs to be addressed. This very simple tool akin to the ESAS tool could be used to screen for spiritual issues. It is adapted from Groves and Klauser (2005) and involves having the person score the following:

Spiritual Pain Scale

Completely Peaceful				General Well-being				Etreme Anxiety	
1	2	3	4	5	6	7	8	9	10

Meaning Pain Scale

Life is filled with meaning and purpose				I feel generally motivated				Life has become meaningless	
1	2	3	4	5	6	7	8	9	10

Forgiveness Pain Score

I feel a deep sense of reconciliation toward myself and others				There are no outstanding issues that are calling for forgiveness in my life				I feel a strong sense of unforgiveness toward myself and/or others	
1	2	3	4	5	6	7	8	9	10

Relatedness Pain Score

I feel a strong sense of connection with the persons and things that matter most to me				The most important areas of my life seem balanced				I feel seriously alienated from someone or something that is important to me.	
1	2	3	4	5	6	7	8	9	10

Hope Pain Scale

I feel hope filled and optimistic				I generally trust what the future holds for me				I am experiencing deep depression and hopelessness	
1	2	3	4	5	6	7	8	9	10

Other tools and accompanying examples of specific questions from Taylor (2010) include:

HOPE

H: Sources of hope: * What gives you hope?

O: Organized religion: * Are you a member of a religious or spiritual community?

P: Personal experience or practice: *What beliefs are most helpful or meaningful?

E: Effects on medical care: *How do your beliefs affect the kind of medical care you would like to receive?

FICA

F: Faith: *What is your faith?

I: Importance/influence: *What importance does your faith have in your life?

C: Community: *Are you part of a religious community?

A: Address: *How would you like me to address these issues in providing care?

SPIRIT

S: Spiritual belief system: *Do you have a formal religious affiliation?

P: Personal spirituality: *In what ways is your spirituality important to you?

I: Integration: *Do you belong to a religious or spiritual community?

R: Ritualized practices and restrictions: *What practices are important to you?

I: Implications for medical care: *Do you have beliefs that will affect medical care?

T: Terminal events planning: *Are there aspects of care at end of life that we should incorporate in your care plan.

Regardless of the assessment tool used, spiritual needs at the end of life need to be explored regularly. The process needs to be determined by members of the interdisciplinary team and documented such that unnecessary repetition is avoided. Re-evaluation is needed to ascertain the extent to which counselling and support is meeting the needs of the person and/or family (Okon 2005).

Interacting with the Individual and Formal/Informal Caregivers

Serious illness forces a person to ponder and perhaps even reappraise the meaning in life and the meaning of life. Meaning has everything to do with relationships, connectedness, and spirituality. While the process of finding meaning involves an inward journey, it also relies on the telling of the story of the journey (Bornman & Brown-Saltzman, 2010).

In order to appreciate the uniqueness and complexity of a person's journey, asking open-ended questions can help the person to tell the story. Open-ended questions begin with how, what, when, who or phrases such as "tell me about". Generally, questions beginning with why are not helpful due to the sense of threat or challenge. (Taylor 2010)

Questions that inquire about the person's feelings or experience are generally welcomed. (Baird 2010) Examples include:

- Are you scared?
- What makes life worth living?
- Is there anything that you haven't done that you need to do?
- What do you hope for?
- What are you most afraid of?
- Is there anything worse than death?
- What are you most proud of in your life?
- Do you have regrets?

Every time a caregiver listens to another person's experience or life story, he or she is involved in spiritual care giving. "Listen for more than words; listen for symbols; listen for where the person places energy; listen for emotion in addition to cognition."(Taylor, 2010).

The person will discover answers and find meaning in life by asking questions and telling his or her story. It is not up to the caregiver to provide answers; he or she can only share thoughts and ideas. Only the person will be able to discover the answers to his or her questions and the meaning of his or her life.

Silence is necessary when listening to a person's spiritual and sacred story and should never be seen as a waste of time. Sometimes when an emotion is experienced, it takes time to find the words to express it; the person needs to take time to collect his or her thoughts. Frequently silence is necessary for new insight to break through. Caregivers must listen for more than words. Silence allows the listener to closely observe behaviours that can convey a message. A caregiver's silence can communicate support, acceptance, and understanding. Silence is a valuable and powerful therapeutic technique that can:

- Encourage a person to talk
- Indicate unconditional acceptance
- Show respect.

Gaining comfort with silence is a skill that can be learned.

Although observations, interactions or assessments of physiologic issues are readily documented, similar information regarding issues in the spiritual domain is less frequently documented.

Merely documenting a religious affiliation and whether the person wishes to have a referral to the spiritual care provider does not adequately indicate a person's spiritual status and need (Taylor, 2006). Spiritual observations and care should be documented for the following reasons:

- To facilitate understanding and awareness of the person's issues

- To emphasize the importance of the holistic approach in hospice palliative care and to meet accreditation standards for holistic care

- To encourage ongoing communication with the person and facilitate continuity of care by enhancing communication among the hospice palliative care team members

In a multi-faith, multi-cultural society like Canada, health care providers must be humble in acknowledging their ignorance of the tenants of many of the world religions. Just as the different Christian denominations have different beliefs and practices, so do other religious traditions. Even within a particular tradition there will be those who are more orthodox in their understanding than others. Although having a cursory understanding of the world's major religious traditions provides team members with a framework for inquiry, remaining open to the variation of religious experience and expression is essential (Taylor 2010). **Cultural and religious sensitivity demands that we never assume but, rather, ask the person or family to provide information about how particular beliefs and practices should be included in the care plan.**

Providing Supportive Care Strategies

The goal of care is to encourage spiritual wholeness and a sense of well being, connectedness, and peace. Exploring and acknowledging one's own deeply held beliefs and values and engaging in personal spiritual questing enables the caregiver to more fully appreciate the centrality of spirituality and / or religion in the lives of many persons and families as they approach death.

When providing spiritual support:

- Respect the beliefs of the individual and the family

- Respond to the individual's spiritual needs according to his or her religious background and belief system. Remember that there are individual sectarian beliefs and practices within each of the major religious traditions

- Share personal beliefs sensitively only if requested

- Do not proselytize or try to convert the person to your beliefs

- Provide whatever the person asks for in terms of spiritual support or contact the spiritual care provider of person's choice

- With permission, engage the person's faith community in providing care

- Observe the person's environment for clues about his or her spiritual/religious inclination. Are there religious pictures, sacred writings or objects on the wall or at the bedside?

Groves et al (2005) offer a variety of traditional healing tools and therapies to support persons who are dying. Most of these strategies have a precedent in the ancient books of the dead and have been tested in contemporary clinical practice.

- Art therapy (e.g. the Sacred Circle or Mandala, doodling, art journals, clay creations, sand painting, death masks) The arts whether music, drama, dance, poetry, drawing or photography may help a person to gain new insight as well as to give expression to ideas and insights.

- Breath work: Begins with a relaxation exercise and then mingles the breath. The anamcara or soul friend synchronizes his or her breathing with the person's breathing

- Dream work is often successful in bringing forth hidden anxieties. Dreams can be recalled, shared, recorded, or drawn. The feelings created in the dream are explored as well as the content. In most cases it is more important to be a dream companion than a dream therapist

- Energy therapies (e.g. gentle exercises / active or passive range of motion, Reiki, therapeutic touch, Tai Chi, massage)

- Touch is a way of sharing intimacy but requires permission from the person. When sensitively and cautiously utilized by caregivers, touch can be very healing. Caregivers need to ensure that couples are provided with the privacy to experience the warmth, tenderness, and expression of love that is conveyed through sexual intimacy (Lamb, 2006)

- Forgiveness exercises (e.g. Life review and forgiveness list, Twelve Step Process, prayers of gratitude which can serve as a spiritual shortcut to forgiveness)

- Guided visualizations (can include healing and assistance from ancestors)

- Healing religious abuse e.g. the abuse suffered by many native Canadians in residential schools and sexual abuse suffered by children who were sexually assaulted by those in positions of authority

- Examining frightening images of a judgmental and wrathful God and comparing such images with those of a loving, nurturing and compassionate God

- Intercessory prayer: As long as intentions are pure, you cannot harm another person with prayer. Everyone has the capacity to be a conduit of loving kindness. Prayer connects one to God but can also connect one to others. Knowing that one is being prayed for by those near and far can be deeply nurturing (Borneman & Brown-Saltzman, 2010)

- Journaling e.g. waking journaling, random journaling, prayer journaling, life geographying (a form of life review based on mapping out life events that occurred within specific time periods), portraits of the soul (adding a picture or doodle to the writing)

- Life review can involve looking at disappointments as well as times of joy and playfulness. Further reflection on themes, may help the person to discover commonalities such as high expectations leading to disappointment. Making a hurt listing; those that the person disappointed and those who disappointed the person can help the person move from disappointment to forgiveness. If the person is willing, arrangements can be made to meet with those on the list with whom closure is important

- Rituals: connectedness may consist of a loving relationship with a Higher Power, a faith community, family and friends as well as oneself. A professional spiritual caregiver (chaplain or community spiritual caregiver) can be a companion on the journey and perform rituals that promote connectedness and peace as well as meet other religious needs. Experiencing a connection to all of creation can be realized by gazing at the sky, the clouds, or a sunset; it can simply be by being outdoors and feeling the wind or breathing the fresh air

- Rituals of release can include the Native American tradition of potlatch (the ceremonial distribution of belongings), giving permission to die, praying a litany of release

- Meditation practices may include centering prayer, davvening practices, lectio divina, metta, breathing meditation, walking meditation, praying a mantra. Meditation can be a powerful act of transcendence. The practice of meditation in the form of prayer, guided imagery, breathing techniques or a mantra allows the person to maintain a sense of control and yet relinquish control (Bornman & Brown-Saltzman, 2006). The relaxation response that is experienced in meditation fosters a sense of peace and calmness

- Music therapy needs to be attuned to the person and not what the caregiver thinks would be helpful. Ask the person or family the type of music that might be meaningful. If person is comatose, watch for signs that would indicate reaction to the music. e.g. restlessness, changes in breathing pattern, frown or relaxation

- Religious rites and sacred writings can be utilized in communion with others from the community or by the person with his or her pastor or soul friend

- Creating a sacred space: A sense of peace can be promoted by paying attention to the environment. A noisy cluttered room may hinder spiritual reflection, while a quiet restful room may assist a person's spiritual exploration and expression. Providing an environment suited to meeting the person's spiritual needs is an important aspect of spiritual care giving. Providing privacy and a moment of honour and focused attention may allow the tears to spill or the anguish to be spoken. When alienation is broken, healing can begin (Bornman & Brown-Saltzman, 2010).

Being present on a consistent basis throughout the process of dying is *primary spiritual care*. The caregiver has an opportunity to provide this care by simply being present; all that is required is to "watch" through the night in the face of suffering, fear, despair, and all the physical, emotional, social, and spiritual trials of dying (Kemp, 2010). Being fully present involves letting go of one's own fears and needs in order to be with the other. Presence may in fact be the greatest gift the caregiver can give to those who are living with life threatening illness (Bornman & Brown-Saltzman, 2010).

Working as a Team

Barriers to providing spiritual care in team members may include feelings of embarrassment, insecurity related to spirituality, or can be the result of personal painful spiritual doubts or struggles (Taylor 2010). Personal philosophy or world view can colour assessment techniques and interpretation. Self awareness on the part of all team members involved in hospice palliative care is necessary if team members are to be comfortable in dealing with other's struggles.

All individuals involved with the person need to share with other team members any disclosures indicative of spiritual pain. Referrals can be made to spiritual care providers or members of the team may be able to assist the team member who has been chosen by the person to be the anamcara or soul friend.

The practice of mercy – of watching through the night – is central to hospice palliative care. The caregiver team has the great privilege of participating in the "watching through the night"(Kemp 2006) Team members contribute to this process by sharing with each other their particular observations, interactions, interventions and outcomes.

There are a number of interventions that require team collaboration, coordination and cooperation.

- Organizing clergy/chaplain visits, worship services or other rituals when physical or other limitations are a barrier to attendance at a place of worship requires team collaboration

- Empowering the dying person to contribute to the wellbeing of others requires team ingenuity. Members of the team offer the person examples of activities that other dying persons have engaged in to benefit others e.g. creating or affirming memories through scrapbooks, audio or video tapes), planning a funeral service or celebration of life, creating a legacy, sharing wisdom, giving away treasured possessions, praying for others, or making a point of reconciling with others

- Fostering and enabling participation in prayer, ritual, and sacred reading activities requires planning on the part of various team members

- Healing music can be provided by a few choir members coming to the home or by providing favourite selections via an audio system at the bedside. Various team members can collaborate in making such interventions a reality.

By being present and witnessing to what is sacred for the person and family, team members indicate that grappling with spiritual issues is normal and valuable as they journey with a progressive illness.

Reference List

Borneman, T.& Brown-Saltzman, K. (2010). Meaning in Illness. In B.R. Ferrell & N. Coyle (Eds), *Textbook of Palliative Nursing*. New York: Oxford University Press.

Baird, P. (2010) Spiritual Care Interventions. In B.R. Ferrell & N. Coyle (Eds), *Textbook of Palliative Nursing*. New York: Oxford University Press.

Ferris, F.D., Balfour, H.M., Bowen, K., Farley, J., Hardwick, M., Lamontagne, C., Lundy, M., Syme, A., West, P. (2002). *A Model to Guide Hospice Palliative Care; Based on National Principles and Norms of Practice*. Ottawa: Canadian Hospice Palliative Care Association.

Groves, R. *Anamcara Project*. Retrieved from http://www.sacredartofliving.com/anamcaraproject. htm February, 2011.

Groves, R., & Klauser, H. (2005) *The American Book of Dying Lessons in Healing Spiritual Pain*. Berkley; Celestial Arts.

Hallenbeck, J. (2003) *Palliative Care Perspectives*. New York: Oxford University Press

Kemp, C. (2010). Spiritual Care Interventions. In B.R. Ferrell & N. Coyle (Eds), *Textbook of Palliative Nursing*. New York: Oxford University Press.

Okon, T. (2005) *Spiritual, Religious and Existential Aspects of Palliative Care. Journal of Palliative Medicine volume 8 number 2* April 2005 pg 392-414

Taylor, E. J. (2010). Spiritual Assessment. In B.R. Ferrell & N. Coyle (Eds), *Textbook of Palliative Nursing*. New York: Oxford University Press.

Wright, L.M. (2005) *Spirituality, Suffering and Illness: Ideas for Healing* Philadelphia: F.A. Davis   Company.

Chapter Eight

Practical

Person and Family

- Demographics

- Culture

- Personal values, beliefs, practices and strengths

- Developmental stage, education, literacy

- Disabilities

Practical

- Activities of daily living (e.g. personal care, household activities)

- Dependents, pets

- Telephone access, transportation

Ferris et al., 2002

Understanding the Fundamentals

Family Roles and Relationships

Understanding the experience of illness for the person and his or her family begins with the concept that the person and his of her family are a "unit of care". Care providers become closely engaged with many different families, as most individuals receiving hospice palliative care are supported by a family. Facing the usual business of living and directly dealing with dying is challenging for all members of the family.

When a family member is facing a life-threatening illness, all members are affected and adjustments in the usual roles and responsibilities within the family result. As disease progresses, the person is less and less able to continue his or her usual recreational activities or to participate in many formerly enjoyed family activities. The person will also be facing the loss of work roles, social roles and usual family roles. A mother may no longer be able to care for her children and instead observes as others take on this role. A husband may be frustrated and concerned as he sees his wife having to complete work in the home that was formerly his responsibility. This inability to fulfill usual roles and responsibilities may threaten a person's sense of worth. Instead of feeling as if he or she is a contributing member to family life or society, the person may come to feel dependent on others or even to feel like a burden. However, it is possible for people who are facing such changes to actually experience personal growth, healing of estranged relationships, and to find new ways or roles to contribute to their family and community. Byock, (2009) reminds us of Freud's definition of mental health as the ability to love and work. When a person has relinquished expectations of being able to work, the capacity to love may be the predominant determinant of a person's health. A person who feels loved and is able to love may express a sense of wellbeing despite the pains of illness, fears of the future and rigors of treatment.

Each family has unique patterns of interaction and coping; and the individual family members have usual roles and responsibilities, formal and informal, that they fulfill. Some family members may need to add care giving and/or additional household duties to the usual roles. Family members have always cared for ill family members but the expectations placed upon caregivers today is much more complicated than in the past (Glass, Cluxton, Rancour, 2010). Family caregivers provide for the needs of most long term and medically complex family members for months and sometimes years. Most of these caregivers are themselves middle aged or older and most are women. Care giving consumes time and money, affects employment, and is associated with depression and thoughts of physician assisted suicide and euthanasia (Lynn, Schuster, Wilkinson & Simon 2008). Carol Levine (1999) is a family caregiver who has focused attention on the abandonment of the chronically ill and their overwhelmed caregivers. In her article, "The Loneliness of the Long-Term Care Giver" she indicates that caregivers want better communication with professionals, education and training, emotional support, and advocacy to obtain needed services for their ill family member and for themselves. They want help in negotiating the system, and they want respite tailored to their needs. She reminds us that family caregivers need support and it should be provided because the health care system cannot manage without them. Another compelling reason to provide adequate support is that caregivers are at risk for mental and physical health problems themselves. Exhausted caregivers become the recipients of care!

Family members may experience feelings of abandonment, anger, and frustration. They need to face their own losses and various family members are often at different points in their grieving process. Each member of the family may have a different way of coping and members are not always able to support one another.

There are some relatively recent developments in Ontario and in Canada which can be of practical and financial help to family caregivers involved in end-of-life care.

Caregiver Assistance

Two types of assistance have been developed to help family members who want to provide care and support to a family member who is gravely ill. One type supports a leave from work; the other type provides benefits for the caregiver.

1. Work Leave

   • An amendment made to the provincial Labour Code now allows a leave of up to eight weeks duration with job protection for the purpose of providing compassionate care to a family member.

2. Compassionate Care Benefit

   • In January 2004, the federal government put into place the Compassionate Care Benefit Program under the Employment Insurance Program. A family member can apply to receive up to six weeks of benefits.

Compassionate care benefits originally were available to care for the following family members:

Child or the child of their spouse or common-law partner;

• Wife/husband or common-law partner;

• Father/mother;

• Father's wife/mother's husband;

• Common-law partner of the father/mother (a conjugal relationship for at least a year)

Effective **June, 2006**, the definition of "family member" has been expanded by the Government of Canada. A family member can now receive compassionate care benefits to provide care or support to the following family members (Government of Canada, 2006):

• Brothers or sisters and stepbrothers and stepsisters

• Grandparents and step grandparents

• Grandchildren and their spouse or common-law partner

• Son-in-law and daughter-in-law, either married or common-law

• Father-in-law and mother-in-law, either married or common-law

• Brother-in-law and sister-in-law, either married or common-law

• Uncle and aunt and their spouse or common-law partner

• Nephew and niece and their spouse or common-law partner

• Current or former foster parents

• Current or former foster children and their spouse or common-law partner

• Current or former wards

• Current or former guardians or tutors and their spouse or common-law partner

A medical certificate from a physician is needed to indicate that a person is gravely ill with a significant risk of death in the next six months (26 weeks). The six weeks of compassionate care benefits can be shared among members of a family. Each family member must apply for and be eligible for these benefits. Individual family members can claim the benefits at any time during the 26-week period, either at the same time or at different times (maximum 6 weeks in total).

For further information visit: www.servicecanada.gc.ca/eng/ei/types/compassionate_care.shtml

Another program that can be of great assistance to families is the Share the Care Program.

The concept is that by inviting friends, acquaintances, neighbours, former colleagues and others to form a support team, the burden of care is lessoned for the primary caregiver and the person who is ill can be provided with many opportunities to enhance quality of life. Practical tasks such meal preparation, shopping, yard work etc. can be delegated to members of the team. Activities that the person enjoys and periods of respite for the primary caregiver can also be organized by the share the care team. The team can be as formal or informal, as small or a large as the person and family wish. Frequently, the family will need support in implementing the concept. There are excellent resources at www.sharethecare.org.

Unfortunately, sick people often resist help and underestimate the extent to which friends and neighbours are willing to help. The person may fear losing control if others get involved and may be concerned about privacy. Family members themselves may also resist help and it may take time to come to the realization that support is needed. When heavy reliance is placed on one or two people, the risk of burnout is high. Primary caregivers need not feel guilty about being honest about their own needs and feelings. They may have to tell the ill person that if they are to continue helping him or her, they will need support. (Capossela & Warnock 2004)

Observing the Individual's Experience

Most changes in roles and responsibilities within the family begin with an ending of life as the family has known it. Davies and Steele (2010) describe the transition of "fading away". The family is required to redefine itself from what used to be to what is now. When capacities are seriously challenged, and persons can no longer do what they want to do, they begin to accept the limitations albeit with great sadness and grief. Feasible alternatives are sought and implemented and new ways of finding meaning and enjoyment are found. The better the person is able to redefine him or herself, the easier it is for spouses and others to provide support, to discuss the changes and to attend to unfinished business. When a parent is able to redefine, children are better able to appreciate that death is a part of life (Davies et al 2010).

Family members who search for meaning frequently re evaluate their goals. Sacrificing today for the sake of a future goal may no longer make sense. They may want to make the best of each day and enjoy the time they have left. Those who don't search for meaning or are unable to find meaning often focus on simply "getting through" or enduring.

Sexuality is a sensitive issue which needs to be addressed in hospice palliative care. "A person's sexual identity can be both altered and compromised during the course of an incurable disease, deleteriously affecting both the identity and the role fulfillment of the affected persons" (Lamb 2006). The ability to give and receive physical love does not evaporate with the diagnosis of a progressive life limiting illness. Matzo (2010) acknowledges the broad complexities of human sexuality and utilizes the Sexual Health Model that identifies ten broad components that are considered essential domains of healthy human sexuality. The components are:

- Talking about sex
- Culture and sexual identity
- Sexual anatomy and functioning
- Sexual health care and safer sex
- Overcoming challenges to sexual health
- Body image
- Masturbation/fantasy
- Positive sexuality
- Intimacy and relationships
- Spirituality and values.

The ability to talk comfortably and explicitly about sexuality, especially one's own sexual values, preferences, attractions, history and behaviours is the cornerstone to sexual health. However, each individual/couple will determine their comfort level with discussions and to what extent physical expressions of love will remain a part of their life. Couples may need assistance from the team and by addressing the topic of sexuality early in the trajectory, sexual issues are legitimized and it will be easier for the couple to voice any concerns as the illness progresses.

Individuals and families rely on the health care team to recognize everyday practical issues that affect their lives. They need guidance and support in working out practical concerns throughout the journey. Sometimes practical issues are the straws that break the camel's back. Lack of support and lack of confidence have been found to be determinants of hospital admissions. Families attribute this breakdown in family coping to lack of support from the health system, fragmentation of services and lack of preplanning. (Davies 2010). Good palliative care is an exercise in anticipation. Monitoring the coping of all members of the family is important in avoiding caregiver burnout.

Interacting with the Individual and Formal/Informal Caregivers

When interacting with the person and his or her family it is important for the caregiver to:

- Recognize that each person and family is unique; the person may have a history of troubled familial relationships, a loosely organized family, or a "tightly knit" family

- Avoid "taking sides" in a family situation, and remain non-judgmental

- Foster communication and understanding between the person and his or her family members

- Resist imposing personal standards and values, and respect cultural and religious differences of the person and his or her family

- Be sensitive to the economic difficulties of the person or his or her family

- Be aware that feelings of anger, grief or depression are unique to each person and manifest differently

- Establish boundaries early with the person and his or her family (i.e. what the formal caregiver is willing/not willing to do)

- Immediately report to a supervisor any suspected abuse of the person

As the formal caregiver engages in a therapeutic encounter with the person and family, it is helpful to understand how to build a comfortable therapeutic relationship. This is a process that begins with the first visit and continues throughout the contact. Some tips for this communication include:

- Sit at the same level as the person

- Say the person's name (only use a first name if given permission)

- Offer the opportunity for privacy and uninterrupted time for unhurried discussion

- Acknowledge that several brief discussions may be better than a single lengthy one

- Observe and respect mood and behaviour

- Be guided by the person about how much contact is comfortable

- Explore background and interests, e.g. the person's preferences in music

- Heaviness, sadness, anger, frustration may need to be acknowledged before any further issues are raised

- Address issues of sexuality by asking questions such as:

  - Some people who have a serious illness are frustrated by the lack of private time with their spouse/sexual partner. How is this experience for you?

  - How often do you have intimate relations with your partner?

- Are you comfortable discussing sexual issues with me? If not, is there someone else on the team that you would feel more comfortable with in discussing any sexual concerns?
- Set boundaries to help the person to feel safe and know what they can and cannot expect from the caregiver
- Respond to opportunities to talk about death
- Be respectful
- Be honest; use gentle truth telling

Introduce the concept of a Share the Care Team when the person is experiencing difficulties with activities of daily living (ADLs) e.g. ambulating, grooming, preparing meals etc. and instrumental activities of daily living (IADLs) e.g. driving, shopping. There may be reluctance to consider the idea of a care team at first as the person may not want to impose upon friends and neighbours. Over time, the person may come to realize that it takes a village to care for a gravely ill or dying person. It may be the family members who recognize the need for more assistance and take the initiative to develop a share the care team.

Supportive Care Strategies

General Guidelines for Caregiver Interventions

Davies and Steele (2010) outline four interventions for formal caregivers to support a person and family members:

1. Maintain hope in the person with a terminal illness and family members

- As families move through the illness, the nature of their hope can change on an ongoing basis. The hope for a cure may change to hope for remission, which may change to hope for comfort, which may change to hope for a peaceful death. Reassure families that everything will be done to ensure the person's comfort. Talking about the past can help to reaffirm good times and the family connections that will continue. Referring to the future beyond the immediate suffering and emotional pain can also sustain hope (i.e. when adult children reassure the ill parent that they will care for the other parent, the person is hopeful that the surviving spouse will be all right). Helping to provide opportunities for the person and family members to carry out cultural practices and rituals may contribute to hope and comfort. Kubler Ross's interviews with dying patients in the 1960s, revealed that even those who were most realistic about their situations left the possibility open for a cure, for some new drug or last minute success in a research project. (Meier et al 2010) Perhaps this hope accounts for the fact that many are willing to undergo significant financial burden and suffering to try an experimental or alternative treatment. That small spark of hope for cure or yet another remission may remain until the last days of life.

2. Involve families in all aspects of care

- With consent from the person, include family members in decision-making and encourage active participation in the physical care of their loved one. Include children in care during the terminal phase and in all activities following the death. The more children are involved in the care (e.g. physical care or decision-making) during the terminal phase, and in the activities following the death, the better able they are to cope with the bereavement process.

3. Offer information

- With the permission of the person, explain to the family what is happening and what they can expect. Doing so provides them with a sense of control. Initiate discussion of relevant issues, such as how the family is torn between caring for their loved one and their own activities.

4. Communicate openly

- Open communication with nurses and other health care workers is often the most important need of families. They need to be informed and have opportunities to ask questions which are answered in terms that they can understand.

Family, friends and even children can help the person and the primary caregiver in many ways. Specific suggestions that can be made to family members and friends include:

- Visit but be aware of signs of fatigue and don't overstay your welcome.

- Offer to do small tasks for the person e.g. walk the dog, return books to the library, take the children to their lessons or on an enjoyable outing.

- Provide opportunities for recreation such as card games, reading aloud, listening to music, reading the newspaper.

- Keep a diary of activities, visits.

- Engage in reminiscence: aspects of history and culture can be transmitted and preserved. Remember that some individuals may be reluctant to reminisce because of painful memories. Respect the reticence.

- If the person is interested, talk about daily activities such as school activities, who you met at the store, what the neighbours are doing.

- Make sure the person is included in conversations.

- Make some meals/treats that the person would enjoy.

- Offer to drive to an appointment or scheduled event or pick up medications or supplies.

- Assist with personal care of the person, if comfortable and the person consents.

- Gather a list of persons who offer to help or are willing to be available. Utilize the list to make a schedule of activities so that everyone doesn't visit the same day or bring treats the same day. Visit www.sharethecare.org for ideas about developing a team to support the person and primary caregiver. There are various tools that can be downloaded to assist with organization of a team.

There are a number of books that can be obtained for families who are providing care to a family member. One such book is A Caregiver's Guide: A handbook about end of life care. The book is available free of charge from the Military and Hospitaller Order of St. Lazarus of Jerusalem and can be obtained through the Canadian Palliative Care Association, local hospice organizations or can be downloaded from http://www.stlazarus.ca/english/projects_pages/palliativecare_pages/caregiversguide.html

Supporting Children: Specific Suggestions for Family Members

Children can be made to feel comfortable when visiting the person, regardless of the setting. They can be supported by:

- Listening to their worries and fears

- Answering questions truthfully with gentleness

- Inviting children to help out in some way e.g. using their art work to decorate the room. Let children be a part of what is happening to the family (i.e. going to get things , letting them help with small tasks such as rubbing the person's feet, hands, Encouraging them to tell the person stories about what is happening in their life

- Letting them know that what is happening is not their fault

- Making sure they know that they will not be left alone

- Always keep lines of communication open

Other ways of providing practical support include:

- Provide education/resources regarding care giving, grief, sexuality
- Be proactive in providing equipment e.g. walker, commode chair, continence products, hospital bed. Notify CCAC when function is declining so that equipment will be there when needed.
- Be specific about what is expected to happen as the disease progresses.

Working as a Team

One of the frustrating aspects of health care for the person is the number of times that the same questions are posed. All caregivers need to have information about the person and family but every member of the team need not ask the same questions. Gathering data regarding the person and family is necessary to provide good palliative care and team members need to determine who will gather the data. There also needs to be a process developed whereby, with the person's permission, all team members have access to information that has been collected.

Practical family information to be collected includes:

- What family members will be involved in care?
- Are there extended family members who need to be kept updated?
- How do family members communicate with one another?
- Who makes decisions in the family and how are they made?
- Are there cultural issues, religious/spiritual practices that would be helpful for caregivers to know?
- How is affection expressed in this family?
- Are there any areas of conflict?
- How is conflict resolved in the family?
- What are the family / household rules that the caregivers should be aware of?
- What are the family concerns?

In terms of practical issues, the following information should be gathered:

- What help does the person need in regard to personal care?
- How comfortable is the person with receiving personal care from others? Who would the person find unacceptable in regard to provision of personal care e.g. child, member of the opposite sex?
- What activities or household duties does the person feel are causing a burden?
- Are there issues with child care, pet care?
- Is transportation an issue?
- Is the person ever left alone? If so, is there need for a system to access help in an emergency e.g. connect care
- Does the person know how to access team members?

The hospice palliative care team members play an important role in assisting the person and family throughout the illness journey. Doing so requires humanity, compassion and warmth in addition to the usual medical, nursing, social, spiritual, and practical care skills. Over and over again, team members are called upon to counsel, educate, train, and support persons and families living with dying. The extent to which the team meets the needs of the person and family ultimately influences how families experience and remember one of life's most profound transitions. (Lynn et al 2008)

Reference List

Byock, I. (2009) Personal Growth and Human Development in Life-Threatening Conditions. In Chochinov, H. & Brietbart, W. (Eds). *Handbook of Psychiatry in Palliative Medicine.* New York: Oxford University Press,

Davies, B., & Steele, R. (2010). Supporting Families in Palliative Care. In B.R. Ferrell & N. Coyle (Eds.). *Textbook of Palliative Nursing.* New York: Oxford University Press.

Ferris, F.D., Balfour, H.M., Bowen, K., Farley, J., Hardwick, M., Lamontagne, C., Lundy, M., Syme, A., & West, P. (2002). *A model to guide hospice palliative care; Based on national principles and norms of practice.* Ottawa: Canadian Hospice Palliative Care Association.

Glass, E., Cluxton, D., & Rancour, P. (2010) Principles of Patient and Family Assessment. In B.R. Ferrell & N. Coyle (Eds.). *Textbook of Palliative Nursing.* New York: Oxford University Press.

Government of Canada (2006). *Compassionate Care Benefits.* Retrieved March 2011 from www.servicecanada.gc.ca/eng/ei/.../compassionate_care.shtml

Kubler Ross, E. Hope. (2010) Cited in Meier, D., Isaacs, S., & Hughes, R. (Eds) *Palliative Care Transforming the Care of Serious Illness.* San Francisco: Jossey-Bass.

Lamb, M. (2006) Sexuality. In B.R. Ferrell & N. Coyle (Eds.). *Textbook of Palliative Nursing.* New York: Oxford University Press.

Levine, C. (2010) The Loneliness of the Long Term Care Giver. Cited in Meier, D., Isaacs, S., & Hughes, R. (Eds) *Palliative Care Transforming the Care of Serious Illness.* San Francisco: Jossey-Bass.

Lynn, J., Lynch Schuster, J., Wilkinson, A., & Noyes Simon, L. (2008). *Improving Care for the End of Life: A sourcebook for health care managers and clinicians.* New York: Oxford University Press.

Matzo, M. (2010) Sexuality. In B.R. Ferrell & N. Coyle (Eds.). *Textbook of Palliative Nursing.* New York: Oxford University Press.

Chapter Nine

Domain: End-of-Life Care and Death Management

End-of-Life Care/Death Management

- Life closure
- Gift giving
- Legacy creation
- Preparation for expected death
- Anticipation and management of physiological changes in the last hours of life
- Rites, rituals
- Pronouncement, certification
- Perideath care of family, handling of body
- Funerals, services

Person and Family

- Demographics
- Culture
- Personal values, beliefs, practices and strengths
- Developmental stage, education, literacy
- Disabilities

Ferris et al., 2002

Understanding the Fundamentals

In western society, peaceful awareness of death is an example of an ideal that is broadly held by those working in hospice palliative care (von Gunten, 2006). Palliative care in the traditional model consisted of end-of-life care but in the current model, palliative care is to be provided throughout the illness trajectory of those with a progressive life limiting illness. Peaceful awareness of death is difficult to achieve unless efforts are made to improve team member's competence in recognizing and communicating issues and engaging the principles of hospice palliative care in the care of the person and family. When palliative care is applied too late in the illness trajectory, the person and family may well have lived for a long period of time with many unresolved issues. It is then difficult to address all the issues in a relatively short period of time in order to achieve a peaceful awareness of death.

Determining when the end-of-life phase in the trajectory of a progressive life limiting illness begins can be challenging. Organizations however do need to determine when persons in their care should be categorized as being at end of life. The question frequently used for classifying individuals for statistical and clinical care purposes is "Would you be surprised if the person died within the next 6 months? " If the health care practitioner would not be surprised, the person is classified as requiring palliative / end-of-life care. Though palliative care ought to begin whenever symptoms of a progressive life limiting illness affect quality of life and comfort, the support provided in the last 6 months of life is important in preparing for the kind of death that the person desires.

As end of life approaches, decisions need to be made. The decisions can range from simple to extremely complex. Ethical principles are frequently taken into consideration in end-of-life decision making.

Ethical Principles include:

- Autonomy: the right of a capable person to determine what may be done to his or her body
- Beneficence: the duty of health care providers to do good
- Non-maleficence: the duty of health care providers to do no harm
- Justice: the fair treatment of individuals as well as equitable distribution of health care resources and dollars

When two or more ethical values apply to a situation but support diverging courses of action, an ethical conflict or dilemma exists. Many organizations employ ethicists to help team members when ethical conflicts arise.

Examples of end of life decisions that may need to be made include:

- extent of family involvement in care giving and decision making
- setting for care: home or in a facility
- caregiver help wanted or needed
- who will make decisions if/when incapacity is determined
- how will limited energy be expended
  - engagement in meaning making, life review, making a will, funeral planning, forgiveness, legacy work etc
  - the withholding or withdrawing of life prolonging interventions e.g. CPR, artificial nutrition, antibiotics
- the timing for withdrawal of life prolonging treatments e.g. cardiac devices, life prolonging medications, ventilation

Friends and /or hospice volunteers are particularly valuable members of the team when the dying person is interested in activities such as life review, legacy work. Volunteers can help the person with activities such as videotaping the person giving a history of the home and precious possessions, writing a life story, and creating memory boxes. These activities require some energy so waiting until the last days to introduce hospice volunteers may jeopardize the fulfilment of such goals.

Friends and volunteers can also be supportive of the family and help them to get away for awhile or get some needed rest. Providing meals or running errands are other concrete ways that they can contribute to care. Since it is not easy for most people to accept help even when it is offered, team members should encourage family caregivers to give their friends an opportunity to help. Consideration can be given to forming a share the care team.

Modern technology with its ability to prolong life along with a philosophy that sees disease as an enemy that must be conquered makes it difficult for physicians and other health care providers to recognize/acknowledge when a person is dying (Head, Ritchie & Smoot, 2005). A particularly toxic chemotherapy regimen or a difficult dialysis treatment can result in symptoms that make the careprovider wonder whether the person is actually dying rather than just experiencing the effects of the treatment. The diagnosis of dying is a combination of science and art. When healthcare professionals are unsure of what to do for dying persons they may simply continue with the treatment they know thereby avoiding the problem of diagnosing dying (Littlewood & Johnson, 2006). Identifying that dying is actually happening allows for appropriate planning, enables informed decisions about end-of-life care and death management to be made, facilitates appropriate use of resources, and the avoidance of futile treatments.

Research using the PPS scores has determined that declining PPS scores are indicative of earlier death and stable PPS scores are consistent with longer survival. Data has demonstrated that with a PPS score of 10%, 50% of persons will die within 24 hours and 97% will die within 7 days. With a PPS score of 30%, 50% of persons will die within 14 days and 98% by 6 months. The Palliative Prognostic Index utilizes the PPS score along with reduced oral intake, presence of edema, dyspnea at rest, and presence of delirium as a tool for determining prognosis. The rate of change in the PPS score is of greater importance than the amount of change. A change in PPS from 50% to 30% is more significant if it happens over 2 days than if it changes over a 4 month period. Personality, the will to live, the extent of disease and the early response to treatment all affect the prognosis. (Downing & Wainwright 2006)

As illness progresses and it becomes apparent that death will almost certainly be the outcome in the not too distant future, the person may become more introspective and wish to withdraw from active engagement in the world. The social circle generally becomes smaller as energy is more and more depleted due to the disease process.

Just as there are developmental landmarks and tasks described for other points along life's journey, there are developmental landmarks and tasks for end-of life.

Byock (2009) describes the developmental landmarks and tasks for the end of life as follows:

Landmarks	Tasks
Sense of completion with worldly affairs	Transfer of financial, legal, and formal social responsibilities.
Sense of completion in relationships with community	Closure of multiple social relationships (employment, commerce, organizational, congregational). Components include: expressions of regret, expressions of forgiveness, acceptance of gratitude and appreciation. Leave taking; the saying of goodbye.
Sense of meaning about one's individual life	Life review; the telling of "one's stories". Transmission of knowledge and wisdom.
Experienced love of self	Self-acknowledgment. Self-forgiveness.
Experienced love of others	Acceptance of worthiness.
Sense of completion in relationships with family and friends	Reconciliation, fullness of communication and closure in each of one's important relationships. Component tasks include: expressions of regret, expressions of forgiveness and acceptance, expressions of gratitude and appreciation, acceptance of gratitude and appreciation, expressions of affection. Leave-taking; the saying of goodbye.
Acceptance of the finality of life - of one's existence as an individual	Acknowledgment of the totality of personal loss represented by one's dying and experience of personal pain of existential loss. Expression of the depth of personal tragedy that dying represents. Emotional withdrawal from worldly affairs and emotional connection with an enduring construct. Acceptance of dependency.
Sense of a new self (personhood) beyond personal loss	Developing self-awareness in the present.
Sense of meaning about life in general	Achieving a sense of awe; recognition of a transcendent realm. Developing/achieving a sense of comfort with chaos.
Surrender to the transcendent, to the unknown - "letting go"	In pursuit of this landmark, the doer and "taskwork" are one. Here, little remains of the ego except the volition to surrender.

In order for individuals to have opportunity to meet the developmental landmarks described by Byock, someone needs to be courageous enough to name the fact that the disease process is one of a progressive nature that will end in death. Exploring these tasks with the person and family is an important role for health care providers. These developmental landmarks and tasks reflect the transition from worldly and social aspects of life to interpersonal aspects, then finally to introspective aspects.

According to the Palliative Performance Scale, a score of 30 indicates that the person has entered the end-of-life stage of the illness. The person will have extensive disease and in terms of function, will be virtually bed bound, unable to engage in activities, and will require total care for all activities of daily living. The person may be fully conscious or may be drowsy with or without confusion. Intake of food and fluids will continue to decrease as the person approaches death. By this point in time it is hoped that most of the tasks outlined by Byock will have been completed and if it is the person's goal to have reached a peaceful awareness of death, that goal will have been accomplished.

Caregivers in hospice palliative care choose to walk closely with the person and family, journeying with them through this important stage of life. By the time the PPS score is 30%, hopefully, formal care givers will have addressed issues in the physical, psychological, social, spiritual, and practical domains. They will be continuing to engage in managing issues and will be assisting with issues of loss and grief for the person as well as the family and in care planning for the end of life. Care givers should be cognizant of what people usually want at the end of life as identified in a frequently quoted study by Singer, Martin & Kelner (1999). The issues identified were:

1. Receiving adequate pain and symptom management
2. Avoiding inappropriate prolongation of dying
3. Achieving a sense of spiritual peace
4. Relieving burden
5. Strengthening relationships with loved ones

David Kuhl (2009) reminds us that only through hearing the stories of those who are experiencing a terminal illness will our understanding and knowledge of human suffering be enhanced. People who are dying are still living! In their quest to know themselves, others and God, they help us to appreciate the fullness of life and challenge us to define our purpose, values and goals.

During the final stage of the dying process two different dynamics are at work in the dying person. On the psychological / spiritual plane, a process of withdrawal and letting go of the material world is taking place. On the physical plane, the body begins its final process of shutting down which results in the systems ceasing to function. In an expected death, these changes generally occur in a progressive fashion and invasive interventions are unnecessary. There are times when incidents that are more distressing, such as extreme dyspnea or a massive hemorrhage, are the final event in the dying process. If such catastrophic episodes are deemed possible based on the person's disease, every effort must be made to prepare the person, the family and the caregivers for the situation.

Sometimes a person who is ready to die may just want it to be over or the family who are exhausted from their vigil may long for the suffering to end. Expressions of a wish to die or requests for help to die must not be ignored. The person who expresses a wish for premature death should be made aware of the team member's duty to report such conversation. Confidentiality needs to be maintained and not everyone on the team needs access to all information. Assessment and management of the underlying reasons for wishing to end life need to be undertaken by the appropriate health care professionals.

One of the reasons for wishing for a premature death is related to the person's sense of being a burden to the family. Simply telling the person that he or she is not a burden is not helpful when it is quite obvious to the person that independence in activities of daily living is virtually lost. Encouraging family members to engage in honest communication is paramount if the best possible solution to the dilemma of dying is to be found. Expressing that yes, care giving is a burden but it is a burden of love or expressing to the dying person that the caregiver is learning and growing because of the experience may be helpful. Additional tips include acknowledging the support that the person has provided to the caregiver in the past or expressing the caregiver's understanding that if circumstances were different, it could be the dying person caring for the caregiver.

Studies have demonstrated that there are significant risks to health and well-being for those assisting in end of life care. Redinbaugh, Baum, Tarbell & Arnold (2003) suggest that the family's ability to accept the fact that the illness will lead to death may determine the amount of strain experienced. It also needs to be acknowledged that not all situations involving end-of-life care are based on a previous relationship of love and kindness.

The final report of the study of Family Caregiver Coping in End-of-Life Cancer Care (2008) determined that those most at risk for negative health outcomes are more likely to be younger females with a low income, who are employed or are taking a paid or unpaid leave from work and who are caring for a parent. The younger women caregivers demonstrated lower levels of resilience and optimism, had greater stress and reported less sense of coherence. These family caregivers also reported feeling less prepared for the care giving role and reported lower levels of family functioning. Those least at risk for negative health outcomes are more likely to be older retired females who are caring for their partner, had higher than average incomes and reported fewer financial worries. They had higher levels of resilience, optimism, sense of coherence and family functioning. These family caregivers also reported low levels of stress and felt more prepared for the care giving role.

For some caregivers, death will be accompanied by feelings of loss and grief, for others, death may bring a sense of relief / liberation. Regardless of the situation, if the needs of both the person and family are identified and addressed in a sensitive way, much unnecessary suffering can be avoided; family distress can be minimized and they can be left with positive memories and a sense of fulfillment.

Observing the Individual's Experience

Ferris, Danilychev & Siegel (2007) identify the following changes and clinical signs of impending death.

Common changes experienced during the dying process	Observable Signs
Fatigue, weakness	Decreasing function, inability to move about in bed, inability to lift the head off the pillow, loss of muscle tone _mottling_
Cutaneous ischemia	Redness over bony prominences, cyanosis, skin breakdown, wounds
Pain	Verbal report if conscious, facial grimacing, tension in forehead, between eyebrows
Decreasing food intake and wasting	Anorexia or loss of appetite, poor intake, weight loss noticeable in temples (loss of muscle and fat)
Inability to close the eyes	Eyelids not closing, whites of eyes showing with or without pupils visible
Altered handling of fluids	Decreasing fluid intake, peripheral edema from hypoalbuminemia, dehydration, dry mucous membranes/conjunctiva of the eyes
Cardiac dysfunction	Faster or slower heartbeat than usual, higher or lower blood pressure than usual, peripheral cooling, peripheral and central cyanosis (bluing of the extremities), mottling of the skin, venous pooling along dependent skin surfaces
Renal failure	Dark concentrated urine, oliguria (urine output less than 400 ml in 24 hours), anuria (urine output less than 50 ml in 24 hours)
Decreasing level of consciousness	Increasing drowsiness, decreased awareness of surroundings, difficulty awakening, lack of response to verbal and tactile stimulation
Decreasing ability to communicate	Decreased concentration, decreased attention, difficulty finding words, use of monosyllabic words, short sentences, delayed or inappropriate responses, lack of verbal responses
Terminal delirium	Early signs of cognitive failure (e.g. confusion, day/night reversal), agitation, restlessness, hallucinations, purposeless repetitive movements, moaning, groaning
Respiratory dysfunction	Shortness of breath, changes in ventilator rate (first increasing then slowing), decreasing tidal volume (volume of gas inhaled and exhaled in one respiratory cycle), abnormal breathing patterns e.g. apnea (breath becomes shallow and there is a period of not breathing), cheyne stokes respirations (breathing becomes shallower and shallower, slower and slower until it stops for a period of time and is followed by progressively stronger and deeper respirations with the cycle being repeated), agonal breathing (infrequent, shallow, ineffective inspirations)
Loss of ability to swallow	Difficulty swallowing, coughing, choking, loss of gag reflex, build up of oral secretions, gurgling, noisy breathing
Loss of sphincter control, urinary retention	Incontinence of urine, involuntary bowel movements, maceration of skin around perineum, perineal infections (e.g. candidiasis)
Other changes	Fever, sweating, bursts of energy just before death occurs (the "golden glow"), aspiration

As the dying person's condition deteriorates, caregiver burden increases. Monitoring the family for signs of exhaustion is important. Signs of stress include:

- Inability to concentrate
- Changes in sleeping and eating patterns
- Irritability and / or anger
- Forgetfulness
- Increased use of alcohol or tobacco or other drugs
- Weight loss or excessive gain
- Activity that is scattered and frantic

Interacting with the Individual and Formal/Informal Caregivers

Every person's life experience and illness journey is unique. Knowledge of the disease process as well as cultural and family norms will help the formal caregiver to sensitively guide the family at this time. The goals and values of the person and family must be respected and all efforts and interventions should reflect those goals and values. This does not prevent professionals from offering recommendations based on knowledge and experience. Caregivers can provide information and accompany the person and family but must always remember that each particular end-of-life journey belongs to the person and family.

Information regarding the dying process, provided in a compassionate and sensitive way assists the family members to support the person and one another. "People who know what to expect have a very different experience of dying and death than do those who are ignorant of the process"(Ferris et al, 2007). Preparing the person and family has the following effects:

- Reduces anxiety and fear
- Increases competence and confidence in providing care
- Increases the sense of value and gifting during the process
- Creates good memories of the experience
- Prepares them for impending losses
- Shifts roles, responsibilities and support systems
- Reduces dependence on health care providers

Ferris, Ferris, Danikycgev & Sicgel (2007) recommend conducting one or more family conferences to convey information, facilitate the development of an effective team, facilitate life closure, support decision making around issues such as CPR, artificial hydration, organ donation, help arrange for rites and rituals, and encourage planning for the funeral or memorial services.

Comparing dying to being born can be a helpful analogy. Just as there is labour involved in being born, there is labour involved in dying (birthing into a different existence whatever that may be for the person). The labour cannot be taken away and it will go on for as long as is required for consciousness or spirit to exit the body.

There are a number of issues that will need to be addressed as death approaches. Taking the time to educate family will help to prepare the family for the death and can reduce the possibility of conflict.

Planning Issues

As death becomes imminent, the plan of care should be reviewed and clarified. It is important to ensure that family caregivers have the equipment, and supplies, and the information, knowledge and skill to manage the various tasks required of them. Being sure that the family have a number to call for guidance and/or support, encouraging them to call at any time of day or night whatever the circumstance and providing a prompt response to such calls is paramount. Clearly reiterating the plan for expected death in the home can prevent panic and inappropriate summoning of emergency medical services. Transitions across health care settings at the end of life are particularly fraught with complications e.g. medical errors, unnecessary tests, lack of continuity. If the goal is to die at home, family members should be reminded that 911 should not be called unless a crisis arises prior to death that can only be managed in an acute care setting. Provide the family with 24/7 access to telephone contact and suggest that the family call the number before calling an ambulance. If an ambulance is called, families need to ensure that paramedics understand the goals of care and are given the DNR Confirmation form. The DNR status as outlined in a plan of treatment and confirmed in a DNRC form should accompany the person to the setting where care will be given. If transfer to hospital due to a crisis is anticipated, a copy of the care plan should be left in the home with instructions for the paramedics to provide the hospital staff with the current plan of care. "Seamless coordination of comprehensive, reliable and readily accessible medical care and supportive services over time and across settings is an essential hallmark of quality of care"(Lynn, Schuster, Wilkinson & Simon 2008).

Other issues that require planning include funerals, burial or cremation, organ donation or donation of the body to a university. The social worker on the team or local funeral director may be called upon for information and resources.

Feeding and Hydration Issues

One of the concerns frequently expressed by family members during the dying process is that the person will starve to death. Explaining that loss of appetite and of the ability to swallow is an expected part of the dying process can relieve caregiver guilt and frustration. Hunger is not commonly experienced by dying persons. The change in a dying person's ability and desire to eat and drink can be particularly difficult for family and loved ones to accept.

As the body systems begin to shut down in the dying process, adding fluids into the person's system can actually increase discomfort rather than relieve it. Forcing oral feeding or fluids can increase the person's distress and can lead to painful choking and aspiration. With increased fluids there is more of a possibility of urinary incontinence leading to more frequent changes to maintain cleanliness and prevent skin breakdown. This additional activity contributes to increased discomfort and caregiver burden. Retained fluid can cause painful swelling throughout the body and can increase lung congestion making breathing more difficult. Tubes and other high tech equipment can be a barrier impeding physical and emotional closeness. There are times, however, when careful administration of artificial fluid may be necessary to control symptoms at end of life.

Tube feedings are not appropriate in the last stages of a person's life. A number of studies have considered the effects of tube feeding at the end of life, specifically with persons in advanced stages of dementia. Tube feeding was not found to be effective in preventing malnutrition, pressure sores, or aspiration pneumonia. Tube feeding did not seem to provide comfort, improve functional status, or extend life. Potential complications related to gastrostomy tubes in the person with dementia include infection and pain at the site, tube leakage/blockage or migration, nausea, vomiting, diarrhea, gastroesophageal reflux, agitation and self-extubation (Li, 2002). The presence of a gastrostomy feeding tube often results in the need to restrain the person as he or she may try to remove the tube. In a 2009 Cochrane review from London, doctors searched for evidence that feeding tube intervention was beneficial. Lead author Elizabeth Sampson, M.D. stated, "We found that there is no research evidence that tube feeding prolongs survival or improves the quality of life for people with advanced dementia," She noted that some studies suggest that tube feeding may have an effect opposite to the desired and actually increase mortality, morbidity and reduce quality of life.

Again using a birth analogy can be helpful. A newborn infant at the beginning of life does not require nourishment until the mother's milk comes in and the infant is sustained for many months with only fluids and then solids are introduced. The reverse process takes place during the dying stage; the person goes from solids to fluids to taking nothing by mouth. This is a natural process. Newborns respond to lullabies and touch, so explore with the person and family ways in which they might convey to one another their deep desire for peace, love and ongoing well-being for one another. Music, massage, and other complementary therapies can be helpful in conveying the feelings of the heart. There are many more ways to nurture than by providing food but because eating is so much a part of nurturing and celebration in most cultures, issues and family conflicts related to feeding frequently arise during the dying process.

Cultural and religious beliefs can impact decision making around feeding and nutrition and can be a source of conflict between the family and the team. Sensitivity and education about burdens and benefits of treatments is important.

Communication Issues

Hearing is believed to be intact until death; families should be made aware of this so that inappropriate conversations do not take place at the bedside of the dying person. The family should be encouraged to engage in conversations during the times that the person is awake and alert. Speaking at the bedside about the physiological changes happening and that the person is dying is not necessarily inappropriate. It may be very helpful for the person to hear what is happening to his or her body. Reminiscing and celebrating the person's life with joy and laughter as well as expressing grief and crying in the presence of the loved one are all appropriate activities at the bedside. Conflicts should be addressed away from the person and as much as possible an environment of tenderness and care should be maintained. Each family will live the dying process in its own way.

The person who is dying may begin to speak of people who have died. Some people close to death appear to be reaching out to someone and may call the name of someone who has died. Be alert for symbolic language such as "I'm going on a trip" or "Help me pack my bags". These may be opportunities to respond with words such as "I know you have to go and I'll miss you" (Morris, 2001). There are many articles and books written about the symbolic language of the dying including Final Gifts by Callanan and Kelley.

Providing Supportive Care Strategies

As the reality of the situation is recognized, hopes change; each moment is precious.

Supporting the person and family in looking back, reviewing life events and milestones can help the person to identify meaning. Education about the dying process for the person, family, and caregivers is very important. Many people have never watched someone die and fear the experience. Sharing information can alleviate some of the fear and distress. Preparation for an expected death includes preparing the family for the changes that accompany the dying process. With this information, family members may be less likely to expect actions to be taken to address changes that are frightening to the inexperienced person but are normal.

Supportive strategies related to all the domains of issues continue to be relevant in the end of life stage. Utilizing the domains of issues as a framework at this end of life stage can prove helpful in ensuring that issues in all domains are addressed. The Cancer Care Ontario Collaborative Care Plans for each stage of the trajectory can be found at www.cancercare.on.ca/toolbox/pallcaretools/. There is an indepth care plan related to end of life. Strategies specific to managing the active dying process (last days and hours) include:

Disease Management Issues/Management

- Address deficits in understanding of disease, possible co-morbidities and prognosis

- Reassess relevance of disease management protocols (e.g. medications, treatments, clinic visits), testing (e.g. BP, glucose testing, goals of care (e.g. comfort or life prolonging interventions) and plan of treatment and make appropriate adjustments

- Establish most responsible physician and ensure caregiver access to 24/7 telephone support

- Facilitate transfer of the plan of care if relocation occurs

Physical Issues/Management

- Pain and other symptoms

- Monitor symptoms (ESAS), reassess pain and symptom management medications and plan for change in route of administration in the event that the person is no longer able to swallow i.e. oral route to rectal, s/c, buccal or transdermal route. Avoid IM route.

- Educate the family caregivers about care provision at this stage.

- Continue to give around the clock medications for pain, dyspnea, nausea as ordered even when the person is comatose. Monitor for signs of drug toxicity (inability to rouse, myoclonus, as organs begin to shut down. Medication dosage or frequency may need to be adjusted.

- Continue to treat constipation. When intake has been nil for 3 days, it is reasonable to reconsider the need for continuing the normal bowel management protocol.

- Inspect mouth daily for crusting, coating, redness, pocketing of food, sores, white patches and dryness. Report findings. Cleanse mouth with toothettes and favourite liquid q1-4 hours as necessary. Moisten oral mucosa q 15 – 30 minutes with artificial saliva. Use muco to loosen crusting and vaseline for dry cracked lips and nasal mucosa. Ensure vaseline does not clog nasal prongs.

- Monitor for ability to close eyelids and for eye discomfort. Use warm compresses bid, artificial tears or saline drops q 15- 30 minutes or a lubricating gel q3-4h. Eyelash reflex is a useful indicator of level of awareness during the dying process.

- Maintain good hygiene and minimize body odours. Moisturize the skin to minimize risk skin tears.

- Manage incontinence with incontinence products. Consider use of indwelling catheter or condom if incident pain is an issue. If diarrhea is an issue, a rectal tube may help to contain the liquid stool, prevent skin maceration and preserve dignity.

- Manage fever with rectal antipyretics or NSAIDs as well as topical cooling with tepid baths or fans.

- Maintain positioning for comfort; utilize special mattresses and overlays as appropriate.

- Use a careful log roll technique to minimize pain on movement. Use a lifter to avoid shearing and attempt to keep the head of the bed less than 30 degrees the majority of the time if possible.

- Reposition q 1-4 hours until last hours and then reposition (as opposed to turning) only as necessary for comfort and cleanliness. As death approaches, the need for turning lessens as the risk of skin breakdown becomes less important (Ferris et al 2007).

- Use comfort measures e.g. massage, heat, repositioning.

- Report observations related to pain or other symptoms to appropriate team members.

Psychological Issues / Management

- Soothing music may be helpful for both the family and person.

- Monitor coping of family caregivers

Social Issues/Management

- Maintain close contact with family members
- Encourage SDM or next of kin to notify all members of family and friends of current condition.
- Determine any cultural preferences regarding handling of the body at the time of death.

Spiritual Issues/Management

- Notify spiritual companions of the impending death.
- Arrange for cultural and religious rituals as desired by person/family
- Provision of care that will meet the goals of the person and family requires that caregivers have knowledge about what would be helpful. Discussion about traditions and rituals that would be meaningful to the family can help team members to create the space, provide the permission and the privacy for special ceremonies to occur.

Practical Issues/Management

- Frequently clarify the goals of care, the futility of life prolonging therapies and the irreversibility of the dying process.
- Arrange for privacy and hospitality in a facility setting.
- Encourage intimacy including curling up in the bed with the person.

End of life Care Issues and Death Management

- Arrange for respite for family as required/requested.
- Encourage family and staff to say goodbye each time they leave the person.
- Encourage family to give permission to the person to let go and to reassure the person that the family will be okay.
- When the ability to swallow is lost, stop all oral fluids to prevent aspiration.
- Manage terminal secretions by starting antimuscarinic medications (e.g. scopolamine, atropine, glychopyrrolate) early and administering them routinely. Postural drainage in a Trendelenburg position may allow gravity to bring secretions into the oropharynx where they can be removed with a sponge. Do not leave the person in this position for more than a few minutes. Educate the family that the person is not drowning or suffocating. The crackling and gurgling noises are caused by movement of air over pooled secretions that build up in the tracheobroncial tree. These noisy respirations are extremely upsetting for families and they need reassurance.
- Confirm pronouncement and certification plan
- Confirm arrangements for care of the body after death including organ or body donation, funeral/cremation.

Loss and Grief Issues/Management

- Assess family members for risk of complicated grief.
- Provide information related to normal grief and bereavement support available through hospice or other agencies.

There are a number of situations that can occur at end-of-life that are more critical and require special consideration.

If seizures are a possibility due to the particular disease process, appropriate medications need to be on hand to manage the situation. Family caregivers need to be made aware of the possibility and be provided with written instructions for management.

If the dying person has an automatic implantable cardioverter defibrillator, following informed consent, arrangements should be made to deactivate the defibrillating pacemaker when the goal of care changes from prolonging life to only comfort. If the decision is made to keep the device active, offer pain relief and a sedative when the device starts delivering shocks in the last days and hours.

If hemorrhage or exsanguination is a possibility, the person and family need to be made aware of the situation and be provided with instructions. Medication to reduce pain or sedate the person should be available and family taught how to administer it. Dark towels/blankets should be on hand if an external hemorrhage is a possibility. The towels or blankets are used to cover the person and absorb the bleeding.

Terminal delirium is an irreversible, acute confusional state that occurs in the last hours or days of life. Up to 85% of patients will develop delirium in the last weeks of life (The Pallium Project 2008). Failure to recognize and treat delirium may result in worsening agitation, myoclonus and seizures. If signs of active dying are not present, health care providers should look for reversible causes e.g. hypoxia, electrolyte imbalance, acidosis, infections, toxin accumulation due to liver or renal failure, adverse effects of medications, disease related factors, and reduced cerebral perfusion. Always check for urinary retention and fecal impaction as these are easily corrected causes of reversible delirium. Delirium towards end of life is one situation in which a trial of artificial hydration may be warranted. Delirium can be hypoactive or hyperactive. Both types involve confusion with the hyperactive type being more difficult for families to witness. Symptoms often come and go and the agitated state (purposeless movements, e.g. pulling blankets on and off, attempting to climb out of bed, sitting up and lying down, tossing and turning) may be interspersed with periods of calm and lucidity. Terminal delirium is often associated with moaning and groaning which can be mistaken as pain. If delirium is mistaken as pain, the situation is often made worse as increases in opioids result in further accumulation of the opioid and its metabolites as the kidneys are shutting down in the dying process. Look for tension across the forehead, furrowing of the eyebrows or facial grimacing in an attempt to distinguish delirium from pain. If these signs are absent, the moaning and groaning is most likely from delirium. For delirium, antipsychotics (e.g. haldol) are the medications of choice. Antipsychotics lower the seizure threshold so at times, both benzodiazepines and antipsychotics are required for an acutely disturbed person. For terminal restlessness, benzodiazepines may be used but there is a risk of paradoxical agitation.

Ferris et al (2007) advise the following supportive strategies:

- attempt to reduce the day/night cycle reversal by using appropriate lighting during the day and maintaining darkness at night
- provide a quiet relaxed atmosphere
- minimize external stimulation
- preferably keep the person in a familiar environment with familiar people
- avoid using restraints

Death Management

At the moment of death, the vital systems within the body cease to function. It is, for many who work in this field, an experience of the sacred. Something of great significance has transpired and formal caregivers are privileged to be a witness. Some family members may be silent, some may cry or wail, others may engage in prayers common to their particular religion. There is no right or wrong way for family members to respond. Extreme grief reactions may require therapeutic interventions by other team members e.g. social worker, psychologist, chaplain, physician.

Clinical signs of death include:

- Absence of vital signs
- Fixed dilated pupils

Other signs include:

- Eyes may be open or closed
- Jaw will relax and the mouth may fall open
- There may be incontinence of urine and stool, leakage of other body fluids

The plan for expected death should be followed. A nurse (RN or RPN) can pronounce or declare that death has occurred when:

- Vital signs have ceased (pulseless at the apex and absent respirations) and the pupils are dilated and fixed
- The death of the person is anticipated by the person, the family and the health team
- The death has been planned for in a written plan (College of Nurses of Ontario, 1999)

A physician must complete a death certificate. The details of the cause of death can be documented on the death certificate by the attending physician prior to the death but the Certificate of Death may not be signed until after death has been pronounced. Nurse Practitioners may certify expected deaths if they have been involved prior to the death. In certain situations, even though the death was expected, the coroner will need to be notified, i.e. every 10th death in a Long Term Care Home.

When the time seems right, begin caring for the person's body with dignity and respect. Follow the wishes of the family, pay particular attention to cultural customs and the protocols of the agency/home. There is generally no need to rush. The general procedure is as follows:

- The family are invited to participate as fully as they wish in any of the post mortem rituals.
- If it is not a coroner's case, tubes and masks can be gently removed. Dressings may be left intact on draining wounds. The removal of these things is a concrete act that makes real the fact that the person is truly dead. It can be shocking to the family so determining readiness to move forward with care of the body is important.
- The body can be washed and the environment tidied. Remember to practise universal precautions related to blood and body fluids. Wounds are covered with waterproof dressings. The dentures can be inserted if appropriate. The body is positioned lying on the back with the head slightly elevated on a pillow. Close the eyes and place a small rolled up towel under the chin if necessary to keep the jaw closed. (McMillan, Peden, Hopdinson & Hycha, 2000)
- Relatives are invited to spend as much time as they wish with the deceased. There is no need to rush and privacy should be provided as desired. Adequate chairs, access to a telephone (in a private area), refreshments are appreciated.
- If it is a death in the community, the funeral home is called when the family is ready.
- The family is empowered to assist with transfer of the body and to make meaningful funeral arrangements.
- Bereavement resources are provided.

Working as a Team

The last days and hours can be an incredibly stressful time for family caregivers. Team members need to keep abreast of any changes in goals of care and communicate effectively with one another in order to avoid giving mixed messages. An important factor in experiencing job satisfaction depends on dealing well with the dying person and family.

The way the team members interact with the dying person will be observed and family members may engage in similar ways. Team members have opportunity to act as coaches and mentors to families and less experienced staff. Sometimes caregivers have talked to family members about the importance of expressing thanks, telling the person how much they are loved, or that the person might need permission to "let go", and yet observe the family at bedside unable to initiate such a conversation. In such instances, a team member can quietly go to the bedside and tell the person about a conversation with family members who spoke of their memories and how much they love and will miss him or her. Similarly, touching the person before and after the death gives the family permission to do so as well. Remember, people live and die in families that have histories and cultures. Generally they approach death in the same way that they approach life but death is often a new experience that requires a coach.

Developing a team philosophy and actively engaging in team building are primary coping mechanisms that help reduce the stress of team members involved in caring for the dying. The need to work through team dynamics and decision-making are tasks crucial to maintaining the energy and spirit required in hospice palliative care work. Vachon and Muller (2009) identify that the best and most effective outcomes are achieved when professionals work together, learn together, engage in clinical audit of outcomes together and generate innovation to ensure progress in practice and service.

In her book, *Beyond all Pain: A Companion for the Suffering and Bereaved* (1983), Cicely Saunders, the founder of the modern hospice movement, compiled some of her favourite quotes. The following is one that speaks to the experience of many who work in hospice palliative care.

I have seen death too often to believe in death.

It is not an ending, but a withdrawal.

As one who finishes a long journey

Stills the motor, turns off the lights,

Steps from his car

And walks up the path to the home that awaits him.

An American Poet

Reference List

Barbus, A.J. (1975). *The dying person's bill of rights.* Retrieved March 2011from http://www.3hc.org/billofrights.html

Byock I. (2009) Personal Growth and Human Development in Life-Threatening Conditions. In Chochinov, H. & Bietbart, W. Eds. *Handbook of Psychiatry in Palliative Medicine.* New York: Oxford University Press.

Downing, G. M., & Wainwright, W. (2006) *Medical Care of the Dying.* Victoria: Victoria Hospice Society

Ferris, F.D., Balfour, H.M., Bowen, K., Farley, J., Hardwick, M., Lamontagne, C., Lundy, M., Syme, A., & West, P. (2002). *A model to guide hospice palliative care; Based on national principles and norms of practice.* Ottawa: Canadian Hospice Palliative Care Association.

Ferris, F., Danikycgev, M., Siegel, A. (2007) Last Hours of Living. In Emanuel, L. & Librach, S.L. (Eds) *Palliative Care Core Skills and Clinical Competencies.* Philadelphia: Saunders Elsevier

Head, B., Ritchie, C.S., & Smoot T.M. (2005). Prognostication in hospice care: can the Palliative Performance Scale help? *Journal of Palliative Medicine.* 8:3. 492-500.

Kuhl, D. (2009) What do Dying People Want? In Chochinov, H. & Bietbart, W. Eds. Handbook of Psychiatry in Palliative Medicine. New York: Oxford University Press.

Li, I. (2002). Feeding Tubes in patients with severe dementia. *American Family Physicians.*65:8. 1605-1610.

Littlewood, C. & Johnson, M. (2006) Care of the patient dying from heart failure. In Johnson, M. & Lehman, R. (Eds) *Heart Failure and Palliative Care; A Team Approach.* Seattle: Radcliffe Publishing Ltd.

Lynn, J., Schuster, J., Wilkinson, A. & Simon, L. (2008) *Improving Care for the End of Life.* New York: Oxford University Press.

Macmillan, K., Peden, J., Hopkinson, J. & Hycha, D. (2000) *A Caregiver's Guide: A handbook about end of life care.* Edmonton: Palliative Care Association of Alberta and the Military and Hospitaller Order of St. Lazarus of Jerusalem.

Morris, V. (2001) *Talking about death won't kill you.* New York: Workman Publishing Company   Inc.

Redinbaugh, E.M., Baum, A., Tarbell, S., & Arnold, R. (2003). End-of-life caregiving: what helps family caregivers cope? *Journal of palliative medicine.* 36:6 901-909.

Sampson E, Candy B, Jones L. (2009) *Enteral tube feeding for older patients with advanced dementia.* London; Cochrane Database of Systematic Reviews 2009, Issue 2.

Saunders, C. (1983). *Beyond all pain; a companion for the suffering and bereaved.* Aylesbury, Bucks: Hazell Watson and Viney Ltd.

Singer, P., Martin, D., & Kelner, M. (1999). Quality End-of-Life care: Patients perspectives. *Journal of the American Medical Association.* 281. 163-168.

Stajduhar, K., Fyles, G., Barwich, D. (2008) Family Caregiver Coping in End-of-Life Cancer Care Final Report July, 2008: Victoria: Centre on Aging and School of Nursing. Retrieved from www.coag.uvic.ca/eolcare/documents/Coping_Report_Final.pdf

The Pallium Project & Pereira, J. (2008) *The Pallium Palliative Pocketbook.* Edmonton: The Pallium Project

Vachon, M. & Muller, M. (2009) Burnout and Symptoms of Stress in Staff Working in Palliative Care. In Chochinov, H. & Breitbart, W. (Eds.), *Handbook of Psychiatry in Palliative Medicine.* New York: Oxford University Press.

Von Gunten, C. (2006) *Ideals and Compromises. Journal of Palliative Medicine Vol 9,* Nu 6 2006 pg 1238-1123

(Watson, Lucas, Hoy and Back 2006

Appendix A: The Dying Person's Bill of Rights

The Dying Person's Bill of Rights
I have the right to be treated as a living human being until I die
I have the right to maintain a sense of hopefulness however changing its focus may be.
I have the right to participate in decisions concerning my care.
I have the right to expect continuing medical and nursing attention even though "cure" goals must be changed to "comfort" goals.
I have the right not to die alone.
I have the right to be free from pain.
I have the right to have my questions answered honestly.
I have the right not to be deceived.
I have the right to have help from and for my family in accepting my death.
I have the right to die in peace and dignity.
I have the right to retain my individuality and not be judged for my decisions which may be contrary to beliefs of others.
I have the right to be cared for by caring, sensitive, knowledgeable people who will attempt to understand my needs and will be able to gain some satisfaction in helping me face my death.
Adapted from Barbus, 1995

Other Rights include:

- The right to express my feelings about my approaching death in my own unique way.
- The right to die in peace and dignity.
- The right to expect that the sanctity of the human body will be respected after death.

Appendix B: A Plan of Care

A Plan of Care (College of Nurses of Ontario, 1999) for an expected death includes:

- Identification of the person and family's cultural and religious beliefs and values about the death and treatment of the body after death
- Identification of whether the family wants to see the body after death (if death occurs in a facility)
- Identification of the family member to contact when the person dies; (if death occurs in a facility)
- Identification of the most appropriate category of provider to contact the family
- Determination of which category of provider will pronounce the death
- Identification of the physician responsible for determining the cause of death and signing the certificate
- A time frame to carry out these activities
- Documentation of the above information in a written plan of care.

Chapter Ten

Loss and Grief

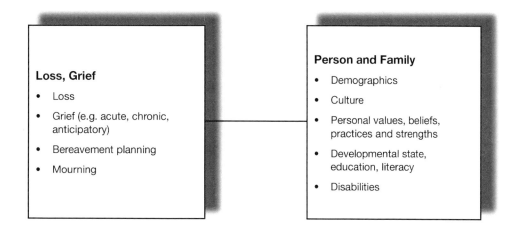

Loss, Grief

- Loss
- Grief (e.g. acute, chronic, anticipatory)
- Bereavement planning
- Mourning

Person and Family

- Demographics
- Culture
- Personal values, beliefs, practices and strengths
- Developmental state, education, literacy
- Disabilities

Ferris et al., 2002

Understanding the Fundamentals

Loss and Grief

Grief is an emotional response to the realized loss of a significant object, person or part of the self and is not first experienced with death. In hospice palliative care, both the person and family will experience grief over the losses that occur all along the illness journey. At each decision point of the journey they will have losses to grieve. For example, with a diagnosis of a life limiting illness, the person will grieve the loss of good health. Changes in body image from surgery or treatment may leave the person grieving the loss of body part or some other aspect of self. As function and independence diminish, the person may be unable to attend an important family function like a wedding or graduation; or family members may see their mother become a different person, unable to fulfill her usual family roles. It is the role of the caregiver to understand grief and support the person and family as they travel on the illness journey.

When the person dies, the family members will make the transition from caregivers to bereaved persons. Death has brought the journey to an end for their loved one but the journey continues for the family. One of the principles of hospice palliative care, the person and family as the unit of care, takes on particular importance following the person's death. The connection with the family does not end for some members of the team. Caregivers need to be well informed about the grieving process to be helpful along the journey; throughout the illness, at the time of death and in bereavement.

Bereavement

Bereavement is described as the state of having experienced the death of a significant other. For example, a woman whose husband has just died is said to be bereaved.

Mourning

Kagawa-Singer (Corless, 2010) describes mourning as "the social customs and cultural practices that follow a death". Mourning is an introspective process that helps a person deal with grief on a conscious and subconscious level. It is also an outward acknowledgment of the death. The rituals of mourning (e.g. funerals, wearing a black armband, burial rites) are an extension of one's social and cultural background.

Factors that Influence Grieving

Some factors that influence the course of a person's grieving in relation to death are:

- Nature of the relationship with the person who died (e.g. mom, dad, child, sibling)
- Perceived nature of the relationship despite what society expects
- Ability or inability to use social support
- Unique characteristics of the bereaved person
- Unique characteristics of the person who died
- Nature of the death (expected, unexpected, violent, suicide)
- Religious beliefs
- Other stresses in the person's life
- Previous experiences with death
- Health of the bereaved individual
- Coping skills of the bereaved

Types of Grief

Knowledge of the different types of grief can prepare caregivers to recognize healthy as well as other types of grief and realize when further assessment and assistance may be indicated.

Anticipatory Grief

Anticipatory grief is experienced before the actual loss occurs. It can begin at the time of a terminal diagnosis. The feelings of helplessness, guilt, anger, denial, fear, confusion and rage can be as intense for the person and family then as the feelings are for the family after the death has occurred. Persons need to be reassured that anticipatory grief is a healthy response to an anticipated death. Grief work can be started when the impact of the impending death is first felt. By preparing for the death, the reality is gradually absorbed. Anticipatory grieving helps the person and family to prepare for the death, attend to unfinished business, participate in life review, resolve conflict, engage in legacy work, and to adapt to changes as they occur. The goal of anticipatory grief is to help the individual cope by discussing details of the crisis before it occurs (Brophy McHale, 2005).

Healthy, Uncomplicated Grief

Grief is the healthy response to any loss or death. It can include physical, emotional, spiritual, behavioural, and cognitive responses. The process of grief is based on the person's perception of the loss. Niemeyer (Coreless, 2010) saw meaning reconstruction as the central process to grief and developed a set of propositions to capture adaptation to loss:

1. Death as an event can validate or invalidate the constructions that form the basis on which we live or it may stand as a novel experience for which we have no constructions.

2. Grief is a personal process, one that is unique, intimate and inextricable from our sense of who we are.

3. Grieving is something we do, not something done to us.

4. Grieving is the act of affirming or reconstructing a personal world of meaning that has been challenged by loss.

5. Feelings have functions and should be understood as signals of the state of our meaning-making efforts.

6. We construct and reconstruct our identities as survivors of loss in negotiation with others.

Complicated Grief

Complicated grief involves the presentation of certain grief-related symptoms at a time beyond that which is considered adaptive (Watson, Lucas, Hoy, Back 2005). Corless (2010) refers to intensive intrusive thoughts, pangs of severe emotion, distressing yearnings, feeling excessively alone and empty, excessively avoiding tasks reminiscent of the deceased, unusual sleep disturbances and maladaptive levels of loss of interest in personal activities.

Risk Factors include:

- Personal
  - Markedly angry, ambivalent or dependent relationship with the bereaved
  - History of multiple loss experiences
  - Mental Health Problems
  - Perceived lack of social support
- Circumstantial
  - Sudden, unexpected death, especially when violent, mutilating or random
  - Death following an excessively long illness
  - Loss of a chid
  - Mourner's perception of the loss as preventable

- Historical
  - Previous experience with complicated grief
  - Insecurity in childhood attachments
- Personality
  - Inability to tolerate extremes of emotional distress
  - Inability to tolerate dependency feelings
  - Self concept, role and value of "being strong"
- Social
  - Socially unspeakable loss (e.g. suicide)
  - Socially neglected loss (e.g. death of an ex-spouse)
  - Absence of social support network

Risk Factors for complicated grief in children include:
- Features of the loss
  - Traumatic
  - Unexpected
- Features of the child
  - History of psychiatric disorder
  - Multiple losses
  - Child less than 5 years
  - Adolescent
- Features of the relationship
  - Ambivalent/conflicted
  - Unsupportive family
  - Death of a father for adolescent boys
  - Death of a mother for very young children
  - Mental illness in a parent

Egan and Arnold (Corless 2006) describe five types of complicated grief.

1. **Chronic** grief is normal grief that continues unchanged for an unusually long time and involves the bereaved person defining him or herself by the experience of the loss e.g. "I am George's widow."

2. **Delayed** grief is experienced when the survivor deliberately avoids feeling his or her grief by avoiding persons or circumstances that are reminders of the loss. The person might work long hours or become overly concerned with others' problems. Resolution comes only after the person takes the time to grieve.

3. **Exaggerated** grief is evidenced by a person who is so devastated by loss that he or she seeks relief by engaging in self destructive behaviours e.g. unsafe sex, alcohol or drug abuse. Safety is a key concern in supporting such individuals as they may attempt suicide.

4. **Masked** grief may be considered when the survivor has an unconscious fear of further loss and distances him or herself from others and rejects attempts to help. Another portrayal of masked grief may involve the person becoming overly dependent on others to the point of straining relationships.

5. **Disenfranchised** grief is grief that cannot be openly acknowledged, publicly mourned, or socially supported. Doka noted that the concept of disenfranchised grief recognizes that societies have sets of norms that attempt to specify who, when, where, how long, and for whom people should grieve (Corless 2006). Examples of those who might experience disenfranchised grief are mistresses or children conceived outside a legally recognized union, homosexual partners, colleagues, friends, ex-wife or ex-husband, step children, families who suffer a miscarriage or still birth. "Grieving in secret is a burden that makes the process more difficult to complete. Disenfranchised grief may also be a harbinger of unresolved grief." (Corless 2010)

Unresolved Grief

Unresolved grief occurs when there is a failure to accomplish the necessary grief work   (Corless, 2010). There are many causes including multiple losses, feelings of guilt, frail   health, lack of support systems, self identity attached to the person who has died,   unfinished business, or lack of closure such as when a person is presumed dead but there is no body.

Unresolved or complicated grief can lead to serious physical, emotional, and psychological issues that can affect the quality of life of the bereaved.

While true psychiatric disorders (e.g. severe depression) following bereavement are reasonably easy to diagnose, it is more difficult to recognize complicated grief in which the pathological nature of the outline the process a person goes through when learning of his or her impending death. However, these stages are actually reactions, emotions and ways of coping that most dying people will experience to some degree. The person is grieving losses at many levels and may react with one or all of the stages Dr. Ross has described. Not all dying persons will go through all of these stages. Important to note is that the reactions can happen at different times, all together, or in no particular order. The stages Dr. Kubler Ross described are as follows:

- Denial – "It can't be true"
- Anger – "Why me?"
- Bargaining – "Maybe I can bargain with God"
- Depression – Accompanies grief and mourning as death approaches.
- Acceptance – Acceptance of the inevitable by the person.

Worden (2002) describes Four Tasks of Mourning and outlines the tasks involved in grief work that may occur simultaneously or in various order. These tasks need to be

completed by persons who are bereaved as they work through their grief, assimilate the loss, invest in new relationships, and go on to develop a new life without the person who has died. For some, this work will mean integrating their experience of loss into a larger acceptance of human mortality. Individuals who have worked through each of these four tasks will sometimes report feeling increased energy and better ability to enjoy their present lives without guilt and fear.

The Four Tasks of Mourning (Worden, 2002)

Task	Description
1. Accept the reality of the loss	• Even when death was expected, there is still a feeling that it did not happen. • This task involves recognizing that the person is dead and will not return. • Death must be accepted on both an intellectual and emotional level. • Traditional rituals, such as funerals, help the bereaved to begin to accept the death as real.
2. To work through the Pain of Grief	• The intensity of the pain and the way it is experienced and expressed is different for everyone. • It is impossible not to experience some amount of pain when someone very close dies. • Friends and family sometimes are uncomfortable with the survivor's pain and may try to interrupt this task. • The bereaved may try to avoid this task by masking the pain through the use of alcohol or drugs, by idealizing the deceased, by avoiding reminders of the deceased, by relocating or quickly getting into a new relationship. • No matter how successful the bereaved person is at avoiding the pain, it eventually will come back again, maybe in the form of depression or when a new loss is experienced.
3. Adjust to an environment in which the deceased is missing	• Adjusting to the new environment is dependent upon the nature of the relationship and what role the deceased played in the relationship. • During this task, grief work focuses on coming to terms with living alone, raising children alone, facing an empty house, managing home maintenance and finances, and caring completely for oneself. • It is important that regression to a state of helplessness, inadequacy or incapacity does not occur during this task. • It takes time and patience to figure out how to take over the roles of the deceased. • It is also during completion of this task that the bereaved tries to make sense of the loss and tries to regain some sense of control over his or her life.
4. Emotionally relocate the deceased and move on with life	• For many, this task is the most challenging to complete. • During this task, the bereaved often finds the ability to invest emotionally in someone or something else. • The deceased is not forgotten, nor are the memories that were shared, but instead, the bereaved finds enjoyment in life again. • In this task, the bereaved do not give up their relationship with the deceased, but find an appropriate place for the deceased person in their emotional life - a place that enables them to go on living effectively in the world. • This task can be hindered by holding on to the past attachment rather than going on and forming new ones. Some people find loss so painful that they make a pact with themselves never to love again. • The deceased are never forgotten or replaced—but remain a part of the bereaved. • The bereaved is not the same person he or she was, and he or she never will be the same again. • With time and grieving, however, the pain will lessen, and the bereaved redefines him or herself.

Corr and Doka (Corless 2010) built on the work of Worden and proposed the following tasks:

1. To share acknowledgement of the reality of death
2. To share the process of working through the pain of grief
3. To reorganize the family system
4. To restructure the family's relationship with the deceased and to reinvest in other relationships and life pursuits

Despite working through grief, it is normal for survivors to hold the deceased in loving memory forever.

Observing the Individual's Experience

By observing the experiences of the person and family, the caregiver will be better able to provide care, resources and referrals that meet needs. Recognizing that grief is an individual and unique experience for each person is critical to providing quality care.

Anticipatory Grief

Anticipatory grief refers to grieving before the actual loss has occurred. It provides time for the completion of 'unfinished business' (e.g. settlement of personal conflicts or finances).

Observable signs of anticipatory grief may include:

• Picturing/imagining (rehearsal of) the death
• Increased concern for the dying person
• Depression (Note: unlike clinical depression, this is reactive ; a deep sadness)
• Attempts to prepare for the aftermath of death
• Avoidance of visiting the dying person

The anticipation of loss may intensify attachment and relationships may get closer and more honest providing treasured memories following death. On the other hand, premature grieving can be problematic if the person is "written off" as already dead. Withdrawal can deprive individuals of opportunities to support one another through the dying process and can lead to the bereaved individual accusing him or herself of having abandoned the person prior to the death. (Zisook, Irwin & Shear, 2009)

Healthy Grief

Physical signs and symptoms of healthy grief (Corless, 2010, Watson, Lucas, Hoy & Back, 2005):

• Dry mouth and throat
• Uncontrolled trembling
• Sleep disturbances
• Loss of appetite
• Stomach pain
• Shortness of breath
• Tight chest
• Weak muscles, lack of energy or fatigue
• Numbness
• Sexual impotency
• Exhaustion

Psychological signs and symptoms of healthy grief

- Deep sadness
- Fleeting visual, tactile, olfactory, auditory hallucinatory experiences
- Anxiety
- Anger

Social signs and symptoms of healthy grief

- Social withdrawal, weeping, startling easily
- Relief
- Shock
- Loneliness
- Yearning

Spiritual signs and symptoms of healthy grief

- Anger at a higher power

Practical signs and symptoms of healthy grief

- Helplessness
- Hypersensitivity to noise
- Difficulty making decisions
- Lack of sense of purpose
- Sense of disorganization

Unhealthy Grief

Signs and symptoms of unhealthy grief include (Corless, 2006):

- Avoiding thoughts or feelings about the death
- Significant preoccupation with the death many months after it occurred
- Large memory gaps
- Flashbacks, hallucinations, or nightmares that occur on a consistent basis
- A continuing, significant disinterest in the activities of daily life
- Calmly and methodically giving away possessions with no emotion and no personal attachment to any of the items. For example, giving away to anyone everything that remotely reminds the survivor of the deceased.
- Feeling consistently guilty about surviving when the loved one died
- Over-idealizing the person who died to the point where it interferes with daily life
- Severe irritability and outbursts of anger toward others in the family, coworkers, friends and/or medical professionals on a consistent basis
- Feeling out of control and unable to cope for an extended period of time
- Using alcohol and/or drugs to keep from experiencing the pain of the grief process
- Detachment and withdrawal from significant others
- Avoiding all relationships for fear another loss will occur

- Flat affect; no emotion, even after the first few weeks following the death

- Continuing tension and insomnia that isn't relieved with relaxation techniques

- Ongoing physical symptoms such as heart palpitations, severe startle reflexes, cold sweats, and breathing difficulties

- The development of new problems related to sleeping, eating, or relaxing that weren't occurring previously

- Talking about or planning suicide

Complicated Grief

Complicated Grief is experienced when the work of grief is too difficult to bear. If any of the following symptoms are present, the person is at risk and may be in need of intensive counselling.

Warning signs of complicated grief may include: (Watson et al 2005)

- Long term functional impairment

- Exaggerated, prolonged and intense grief reactions

- Significant neglect of self-care

- Frequent talking about loss

- Idealization of the deceased

- Impulsive decision making or loss of decision-making power beyond the initial phase of grief

- Major personality changes

- Onset of new chronic health problems

- Mental disorders e.g. drug or alcohol dependency, depression (as diagnosed by a physician, feelings or expressions of suicide

- Post traumatic stress disorder-like symptoms e.g. recurring nightmares, flashbacks, sleep problems, trouble concentrating, hypervigilance, avoidance of people places and experiences related to the stress

Children and Grief

Death is a reality that children can learn to live with. Even before the death of a close family member occurs, parents can begin to introduce the idea of death as a part of everyday life. The nightly news, a trip past the cemetery, or a dead plant or bird may spark conversation about death.

One feature of grief demonstrated by most children is that they do not sustain grief over continuing periods of time, but tend rather to dip in and out of their grief - jumping in and out of puddles, rather than wading through the river of grief. Children will learn about grief, and expressing grief, from the adults around them and should be allowed to express their grief in their own way, be it through play, artwork, or acting.

The following chart outlines the various reactions to grief a child may experience at different ages.

Grief: Infants to Teens (Davies and Jin 2006, Watson et al. 2005)

Age	Characteristics	View of Death and Response
Newborn -6 months	• Basic needs must be met • Cries if needs aren't met • Needs emotional and physical closeness of a consistent caregiver • Views caregiver as source of comfort and all needs fulfillment • Developing trust	• No concept of death • Can sense disruption in routine

6 months to 2 years	• Begins to individuate
	
	• Remembers the face of the caregiver when absent
	
	• Demonstrates full range of emotions
	
	• Identifies caregiver as source of good feelings and interactions
		• May see death as reversible
		
		• Experiences true grief
		  - only to death of significant person in child's life
		  - screams, panics, withdraws, becomes disinterested in food, toys, activities
		  - reacts in concert with distress experienced by caregiver
		  - no control over feelings and responses
		  - anticipate regressive behaviour

2 to 5 years	• Egocentric • Cause – effect not understood • Developing conscience • Attributes life to objects • Feelings expressed mostly by behaviours • Can recall events from the past	• Sees death like sleep, that is, reversible • Has a sense of loss • Curiosity, questioning • Believes in magical causes • Anticipate regression, clinging • Aggressive behaviour is common • Worry about who will care for them
5-9 years	• Attributes life to things that move • May fear the dark • Begin to develop intellect • Begin to relate cause and effect • Understand consequences • Literal, concrete • Decreasing fantasy life, increasing control of feelings	• Begin to see death as irreversible, death is final and frightening • Personify death as ghosts and bogeymen; fear being alone • Interested in biological aspects of life and death • May see death as punishment; may feel responsible • Problems concentrating on tasks • May deny or hide feelings • Vulnerable, fear being alone, worry that family members will die • Developmental delays or regression to previous developmental stage • Fighting and angry behaviour both at school and at home

Age	Characteristics	View of Death and Response
9-12 years	• Individuation outside the home • Identify with peer group but need family attachment • Understand life processes • Can verbalize feeling • Begin to physically mature	• Everyone will die, sense of own mortality • Death is permanent • Strong emotional reaction • Anger and aggression at many people including the person who died • May somaticize e.g. headaches, stomach aches, trouble sleeping • May intellectualize or have morbid preoccupation with death • May experience loyalty conflicts-between friends and family • School work may be neglected or done poorly • May isolate themselves
Teenage years	• Physical maturation continues • Need peer approval • Engage in search for meaning and purpose in life • Attempting to develop a personal identity	• Death is real but will not happen to me! • They may feel that their deep and powerful emotions are not experienced by anyone else • May experience wide mood swings, depression, extreme sadness, loneliness, anger, hostility • May cover up feelings with sarcasm or joking • May have identity confusion -"Now that my dad is dead, I must be the man in the house" • May prefer peers over family members • May test limits • May experiment with (or increase use of) alcohol and /or drugs • May become sexually active • May withdraw from friends and family • Ability with school work may decrease

As the child grows and develops, certain life tasks need to be accomplished. Through the accomplishment of these life tasks and through life experiences, a person acquires skills that determine how he or she will react to different events, including the death of a loved one or his or her own impending death. Since every person has unique life experiences and skills, caregivers will observe many different grief reactions. There is no right or wrong way to grieve.

Interacting with the Individual, Formal/Informal Caregivers

There are many factors which influence how families and individuals cope with death, dying, and loss. To ensure the best possible care for the family it is important for the caregiver to understand how the family copes. This understanding should drive the interaction and effective communication with the family.

- Some of the factors that may affect how families interact with care providers and cope with the palliative experience are:
- Past death experiences, past grief experiences
- Deceased person's role in family (e.g. wage earner, primary homemaker)
- Seriousness and length of illness e.g. prolonged illness is emotionally and financially taxing, creates guilt
- Presence of family and outside social support
- Financial situation
- Cultural differences (e.g. willingness to accept help, expression of emotions)
- Relationship to the deceased
- Age of the deceased
- Age of the family member; children grieve differently than adults
- Coping mechanisms of individuals & family
- Health conditions of family members
- Gender; men & women grieve in different ways
- Nature of the death
- Social value of relationship to the deceased (e.g. death of a lover in a extramarital affair, miscarried or aborted fetus)

REMEMBER!

- Grief is a natural and healthy response to any loss. Every person grieves in a different way, and that way is unique. The caregiver needs to accept the uniqueness of each survivor – where he or she is in the grief process and what helps that particular person.

- Grief is a healthy process that must be done to enable the bereaved to live in a world without the loved one. There is no right or wrong way to grieve, but it must be done.

- Children may do poorly in managing their grief if they are not allowed to express their grief in ways that are healthy for them.

- The pain changes from the acute pain experienced when the loss initially occurred but grieving is never really over. Individuals will experience moments and times when an occasion or object revives feelings of loss, as if it just happened yesterday.

Providing Supportive Care Strategies

There are many different kinds of supportive care strategies for a grieving person or family. This section is organized accordingly:

1. Supportive care strategies prior to the death

2. Supportive care strategies following the death

3. Supportive care strategies specifically for children

Supportive Care Strategies for the Family Prior to the Death

When someone in a family is diagnosed with a terminal illness, everyone begins to grieve. This anticipatory grief process can be confusing and challenging. On the one hand, family members are attending to the needs of the ill person and maintaining involvement with him or her. On the other hand, they may begin to invest emotional energy into planning for life after the person dies.

Formal caregivers can help to ease some of the strain that family members feel by being supportive in ways that help the family members to cope. The following chart describes some issues that family members may have to deal with before the death of their loved one and some supportive care strategies that the caregiver can suggest.

Issue	Supportive Care Strategy
Fluctuating from denial to acceptance of the illness and death.	Some denial of reality is healthy and necessary for a family to function. It allows them to take in information at a more tolerable pace, and gives them a break from the emotional stress of a situation. Acceptance may not necessarily bring peace. Health care providers need to accept the family members regardless of the coping strategy being utilized. An attitude that hopes for the best and plans for the worst is most often helpful.
Establishing a relationship with health professionals.	A family may need to learn how to be assertive and how to deal with frustration constructively. Having the family keep a journal of questions and concerns and providing consistent answers can help avoid confusion and conflict. Family and caregiver conferences can help to reduce anxiety by opening communication lines and providing timely information.
Meeting the needs of the dying person.	As the illness progresses, the person's physical and emotional needs will change. Family members can be counselled to give the person as much independence and control as possible for as long as possible. Keeping the lines of communication open and frequently assessing the needs of all family members can help to keep the plan on track. It is important to avoid placing too much burden on any one person.
Maintaining a functional family unit.	When someone is ill, it means that everyone takes on new roles and responsibilities. At the same time, it is important to maintain some of the normal family routines in order to give some sense of security in the midst of chaos. Encouraging family members to take time to care for themselves and one another is important .The wisdom of the dying person can be transmitted to others in a variety of ways. Sharing knowledge maintains dignity and allows the person to continue to contribute to the family.
Living with the emotions of anticipatory grief.	Throughout the journey, both the person and family experience intense swings in emotion. Having information about these feelings and being aware of the normalcy of such reactions will help relieve feelings of guilt. It is important to communicate with one another but there may be things that each member of the family will prefer to discuss with someone outside the family. Soul friends or hospice volunteers are extremely valuable resources for both the person and individual family members.

Issue	Supportive Care Strategy
Dealing with people outside the family.	Family members may have little energy at this time for outside relationships and may find that other's reactions are unpredictable. For example, friends avoid the sick person and may not understand what the person and family are going through. It is natural to resent others' stability and good fortune. Setting up a Share the Care team may assist in bringing friends together with a common purpose in support of the family.
Anticipating the family's new reality after the death.	It is impossible to predict the future. Estate planning, dealing with different kinds of unfinished business, and building in emotional supports are things that can help people to prepare. Reassure the family members that they are doing the best that they can in the circumstances.
Finding appropriate hope.	What a family hopes for throughout the illness trajectory often changes. Providing accurate and consistent information will assist in decision making and prioritizing goals. As the disease progresses, treatment goals aimed at prolonging life are often changed to goals aimed at comfort. Helping the person and family adjust to a focus on comfort, can lead to acceptance of the inevitability of death.
Allowing the dying person to be at risk.	Allowing the dying person independence and control may sometimes mean refusal to take medications or accept personal help. Family members and health care providers may have difficulty allowing the person to be at risk. As long as the person's choices do not place others at risk, the person's informed decisions must be honoured. Health care providers have an obligation to provide information so that decisions are informed.
Making decisions for the dying person.	There may come a time when the person is unable to make any clear decisions. Prior discussions of the person's goals, values and wishes will help substitute decision makers to make decisions that represent the person's goals and best interests. Health care providers play an important role in encouraging advance care planning and discussions about goals, values and wishes as well as the role of the substitute decision maker.
Care for the caregiver.	When members of the family are focused on caring for the dying person, they may neglect their own health needs. Encouraging them to build in time for self care is crucial. Providers should encourage recognition of caregiver needs - physical, emotional and spiritual – and offer information about strategies to reduce stress.

Supportive Care Strategies Following the Death

There are many ways a caregiver can support family members to deal with grief and loss. Some general tips a caregiver can share with the family include:

- Get adequate sleep; if sleep is not possible attempt to rest and relax, listen to soothing music
- Eat balanced meals; several small meals and snacks with healthy food choices may be easier than trying to eat 3 larger meals
- Drink lots of water
- Exercise; a short walk is better than no walk
- Cry as often as needed
- Reach out for help: reaching out is not a sign of weakness but rather a sign strength and insight
- Consider joining a support group
- If possible, avoid making any major changes for the first year after the death
- Plan ahead for special, potentially challenging occasions such as birthdays, holidays, weddings, etc.

- Avoid use of potentially harmful substances such as tobacco, drugs and alcohol; they only mask the grief

- Attend to the personal belongings of the dead loved one when ready; there is no specific time frame for accomplishing this task.

Grief rituals are another strategy that can help the family deal with the death of a loved one. The value of creating "grief rituals" is in promoting a sense of tenderness, thanksgiving for the relationship, forgiveness, peace and acceptance. Healing can often be achieved through rituals. Too often, bereaved persons feel they must "hold on" to the pain in order to be faithful to the loved one. It is important for the bereaved either individually as a family to create personal rituals that have meaning and significance. Refer to Appendix B for examples of rituals.

Grief rituals are an important supportive care strategy that can be repeated day after day, week after week or year after year. The funeral, celebration of life or memorial service is an example of a ritual that frequently marks in a social way the letting go of the person after death. See Appendix B for examples of grief rituals.

There are many reasons for having funerals/ rituals to mark the death of a loved one and regardless of the culture, those reasons tend to be consistent. According to Rando (1991), funerals/ death rituals:

- Confirm and reinforce the reality of the death

- Assist in the acknowledgement and expression of feelings of loss

- Offer the bereaved an opportunity to express their feelings

- Stimulate the recollection of the deceased loved one, which is a necessary part of grief

- Assist the bereaved to begin to accommodate to the changed relationship between themselves and their deceased loved one

- Validate the life of the deceased

- Allow for input from family and friends that serves as a living memorial and helps to form an integrated image of the loved one

- Allow family and friends to give the bereaved person(s) vital social support

- Begin the process of reintegrating the bereaved person back into society with a new identity

- Provide meaningful structured activities to counter the loss of predictability and order that frequently accompanies the death of a loved one

Supportive Care Strategies Specifically for Children

Supportive care strategies for children dealing with grief and loss may look a bit different than those for adults. Include the child in remembrance rituals, recognize and support the child's unique style and pace through grief, and expect periodic returns to grieving at significant transitions in the child's life. (Victoria Hospice Bereavement Program) Below are some practical supportive care guidelines that a caregiver can share with a family to help children cope with the death of someone close to them (Davies, Limbo and Jin, 2006).

Age	Supportive Strategies
Birth to 6 months	• Progressively disengage the child from primary caregiver if possible • Introduce new primary caregiver • Nurture and comfort • Anticipate and provide for physical and emotional needs • Maintain routines
6 months to 2 years	• Provide continual support and comfort • Avoid separation from significant others • Maintain close physical and emotional connection to significant others • Maintain daily structure and schedule of routine activities • Support caregiver to reduce distress and maintain a stable environment • Acknowledge sadness that loved one will not return- offer comfort
2-5 years	• Remind the child that loved one will not return • Reassure the child that he or she is not to blame • Give realistic information • Answer questions honestly • Involve child in farewell ceremonies • Keep home environment stable and structured • Help put words to feelings; reassure and comfort • Reassure the child about who will take care of them • Provide ways to remember the loved one • Create opportunities for play • Be a consistent and nurturing presence • Do not scold the child for any regressive behaviour- be patient – this is the child's way of coping
5-9 years	• Give clear and realistic information • Include children in funeral ceremonies if they choose. • Give permission to express feelings and provide opportunities • Reduce guilt by providing factual information • Provide structure for the child. Don't give the child too many choices at first, gradually introduce more choices • Encourage the child to talk of feelings through words, play or drawings • Notify the school for additional support
9-12 years	Provide unambiguous information Provide opportunities to express self and feelings Encourage outside relationships with trustworthy mentors Constantly reassure with words and presence Talk regularly to the teachers at school Maintain a constant routine Provide appropriate ways to work out anger and aggression
Teenager	• Dispel fears about physical concerns • Provide outlets for energy and strong feelings (recreation, sports, music) • Create times for communication • Provide mentorship and direction • Honestly answer all questions • Set clear limits and fair expectations • Ask family and friends for support • Seek outside counselling/support groups for the teenager/family

*See **Appendix C** for more information related to supporting children.*

Support for the Bereaved

There are different types of support available through which the bereaved can receive assistance with their grief work. Some persons will benefit from one-to-one assistance; others may respond better to a group setting.

Self Help

Grief can be a very private and profound process. This is a time when the bereaved person will need the support of compassionate and empathetic friends and family. Many self help strategies/complementary therapies such as art, yoga, meditation, massage, may be found helpful. Reading about how others in similar situations coped with grief can also provide insights.

Grief Companions/Hospice Volunteers

Grief companions do not attempt to change the bereaved person's perceptions or attitudes. They encourage the bereaved to work through the grieving process as a natural process that is necessary in order for the bereaved to learn to live with his or her grief. Often times the bereaved person will have been seen by a grief companion for a few sessions and will then join a grief support group for further support.

Support Groups

A support group involves persons who are bereaved sharing their grief stories. In the telling of their stories, they are affirmed that the emotions they are feeling are for the most part normal and healthy. Group members can provide encouragement, information, and practical suggestions to cope with each other's grief. Grief support groups frequently meet for exercise or for social outings and often long term friendships are created.

Professional Assistance

At times a person may become "stuck" in his or her grief. As discussed in this chapter, grief may become complicated for many reasons. A person who experiences complicated grief should seek professional therapy. A professional therapist will attempt to intervene and work with the bereaved to identify and work through conflicts that are preventing the bereaved from living successfully with his or her grief. The therapist needs to have in-depth knowledge of personality patterning and psychodynamics.

Working as a Team

Persons and families living with life limiting illness and the associated loss and grief require the support and skills provided through the diverse talents found in an interdisciplinary team. The team includes the person and family who share their reaction to the illness and their ability to cope. No one member of the team is any more important than another as they are all working towards a common goal.

The physician's primary responsibility is to manage the disease process and control the person's pain and other symptoms. These symptoms must be controlled before any end-of-life grief work can begin (Brophy McHale 2005).

The nurse on the team helps the family cope with the effects of the illness. The role of the nurse in hospice palliative care is further developed in the Comprehensive Advanced Palliative Care Education Program for nurses (CAPCE). Nurses establish therapeutic relationships with families and engage in countless encounters in which they assess, share information, support decision making, plan care, deliver care and confirm that goals are being met and that the person and family are satisfied with the care.

Social Work brings skills that aid in the empowering the person and family to identify and express their needs and goals. By focusing on the effects of life limiting illness on the family system and engaging in honest communication, fear and anguish can be reduced. Social workers are invaluable in helping persons and family members cope with ever increasing losses and changing circumstances along the illness trajectory. They also provide practical resources, information, and referral related to practical, financial, and legal issues.

Chaplaincy can assist persons and families to find meaning and purpose in illness and death. Meaningful end-of-life rituals can be a source of support and encouragement as the person and family face the ultimate loss. Dealing with issues of regret and guilt can promote a peaceful letting go. Remember that denominational clergy, parish nurses, traditional healers, soul friends, spiritual advisors and others may be included under chaplaincy.

Personal Support Workers are in frequent and close contact with the person and family. This close contact provides an opportunity to get to know who each member is as a person. This relationship allows early recognition of changing symptoms and needs. By reporting observations, PSWs are paramount in promoting timely interventions by other team members. PSWs support compliance with the plan of care by reinforcing information provided by the professional members of the team. They support the person and family through their empathic and compassionate care as the family cope with the losses they encounter along the trajectory.

Hospice Volunteers are the team members who act as companions on the journey and bring opportunities to enhance quality of life to the person and family. They come from all walks of life and due to the serious nature of the work are carefully chosen to work with vulnerable people. Volunteers are screened, trained and then supported as they accompany families in the dying process. Volunteer matches are made by considering the skills, talents and desires of the volunteer with the needs and social interests of the person and family. These invaluable members of the team are able to follow the survivors through bereavement.

Palliative care over the years has borrowed ideas, values and techniques from various disciplines and adapted them in the care of the dying. Disciplines such as medicine and nursing have become core parts of the specialist team whereas other professional and paraprofessional disciplines have been called upon on an as needed basis. Increasingly allied health care providers have seen the need to evolve the palliative care specialty within their own disciplines. Because so many life limiting illnesses have a long trajectory, rehabilitation techniques are required to maximize the person's potential after each specific loss.

Occupational therapy can help the person throughout the journey as they move from being totally independent to being completely dependent. The chaotic feelings that accompany the losses along the trajectory are the result of an assault on self esteem. Anger, resentment, bitterness and hostility are energy wasting. OTs can help the individual to identify as well as to analyse their feelings and reactions. They can redirect the person toward an attitude of positivism and control.

Nutritional Therapy is of great value along the journey as goals change in relation to disease progression. The dietician can offer advice related to loss of appetite and other changes such as mouth sores, diarrhea, nausea and vomiting, and changes in taste related to the disease and / or its treatment. Addressing such issues ultimately supports the person in the grieving process related to the many losses experienced over time. At end of life, the dietician supports the team in helping the family to understand that loss of appetite is a normal part of the dying process. The benefit of artificial nutrition and hydration needs to be weighed against the burdens and risks. This information from a dietician may help to relieve the family of any guilt surrounding the issues of feeding.

Physiotherapy is aimed at reducing the degree to which disabilities caused by the disease or its treatment interferes with everyday life. The person who has become dependent due to loss of mobility and function with the assistance of the physiotherapist may be able to regain some sense of control as well as enhanced comfort.

Speech language therapy can be helpful when losses related to speech and cognition are experienced. They can offer advice to the team including the person and family related to communication strategies. In addition, they can offer advice around feeding when the ability to swallow is diminishing.

Clinical psychology is concerned with the wellbeing of the whole team. Experiencing loss through death is one of the most stressful events in life. Psychologists have the skills to encourage expression of thoughts and emotions. Through counselling and skilled communication they help the person, family members and other team members to cope. The DSM 5 edition of the American Psychiatric Association's (APA) Diagnostic and Statistical Manual of Mental Disorders (DSM) is due for publication in 2013 and is currently in consultation, planning and preparation. In the DSM 4 edition, the bereaved are excluded when diagnosing a major depressive disorder. There is considerable discussion around the issue of including bereavement due to a fear that healthy grief will become a medical issue. Pies and Zizook (2011), though they agree with the exclusion, believe that too little attention has been paid to the features that distinguish healthy grief and bereavement from psychopathological states, such as complicated grief or major depressive disorder. In healthy grief and bereavement, the person maintains emotional connection with others; believes that the grief will some day end; maintains self-esteem; and experiences positive feelings and memories along with painful ones. If guilt is present, it is related to "letting down" the deceased person, rather than on being "worthless" or useless. Loss of pleasure is related to longing for the deceased loved one, as opposed to the pervasive anhedonia (loss of pleasure) often seen in severe depressions. Suicidal feelings are related to longing for reunion with the deceased rather than to thoughts of not deserving to live. The person is capable of being "consoled" by friends, family, music, books etc.

In severe depression, the person tends to be extremely "self-focused"; feels outcast or alienated from friends and loved ones; has the sense that the grief will "never end"; experiences profound self-loathing and guilt; experiences few if any positive feelings or memories; and is often inconsolable.

Hopefully by including bereavement as a risk factor for a major depression a "medicalization" of grief will not ensue. Rather, it may encourage team members who observe the signs of potentially serious depressive illness during bereavement to refer the person for further help. All health care professionals need to be astute in observing, assessing, sharing information about grief in order to make the grief process as healthy as possible. When treating the bereaved, premature prescription of antidepressants (eg, within the first week of depression) should be avoided with consideration given to grief counselling or psychotherapy as the first-line treatment for short-lived, mild-to-moderate depression.

Reference List

Corless, I. (2006/2010). Bereavement. In B.R. Ferrell & N. Coyle (Eds.). *Textbook of Palliative Nursing.* New York: Oxford University Press.

Brophy McHale, H. (2005) *Grief and Bereavement.* In Kuebler, K., Davis, M. & Moore, C. (Eds) Palliative Practices An Interdisciplinary Approach St. Louis: Elsevier Mosley

Davies, B., Limbo, R. & Jin, J. (2010) *Grief and Bereavement in Pediatric Palliative Care.* In B.R. Ferrell & N. Coyle (Eds.). *Textbook of Palliative Nursing.* New York: Oxford University Press.

Ferris, F.D., Balfour, H.M., Bowen, K., Farley, J., Hardwick, M., Lamontagne, C., Lundy, M., Syme, A., West, P. (2002). *A Model to Guide Hospice Palliative Care; Based on National Principles and Norms of Practice.* Ottawa: Canadian Hospice Palliative Care Assoion.

Kubler-Ross, E. (1969). *On death and dying.* New York: Macmillan Publishing Company.

Pies, R., & Zizook, S. (2011). *Depression or Bereavement? Defining the Distinction: The Disagreement.* Retrieved from www.medscape.com/article/740333_2 May 2011

Rando, T. (1991) *How To Go On Living when Someone You Love Dies.* New York: Bantam Books.

Victoria Hospice Bereavement Program (2011) Retrieved from www.victoriahospice.org/sites/ default/files/imce/VicHospChildrenTeenGrief.pdf

Watson, M., Lucas, C., Hoy, A., Black, I. (2005). *Oxford Handbook of Palliative Care.* Oxford New York: Oxford University Press.

Worden, W.(2002). *Grief Counselling and Grief Therapy-A Handbook for Mental Health Professionals.* New York: Springer Publishing Company.

Wolfelt, A.(2011). *Helping Dispel 5 Common Myths About Grief.* Retrieved from http://www. centerforloss.com/articles.php?file=helping7.php March 31 2011

Zisook, S., Irwin, S. Shear, M.K. (2009). *Understanding and managing bereavement in palliative care.* In H. Chochinov & W. Brietbart (Eds.). *Handbook of psychiatry in palliative care.* New York: Oxford University Press.

Appendix A: Helping Dispel 5 Common Myths About Grief (Wolfelt, 2011)

Myth # 1: Grief and mourning are the same experience.

Most people tend to use the words grief and mourning interchangeably. However, there is an important distinction between them. We have learned that people move toward healing not by just grieving, but through mourning. Simply stated, *grief* is the internal thoughts and feelings we experience when someone we love dies. *Mourning,* on the other hand, is taking the internal experience of grief and expressing it outside ourselves. In reality, many people in our culture grieve, but they do not mourn. Instead of being encouraged to express their grief outwardly, they are often greeted with messages such as "carry on," "keep your chin up," and "keep busy." So, they end up grieving within themselves in isolation, instead of mourning outside of themselves in the presence of loving companions.

Myth #2: There is a predictable and orderly progression to the experience of grief.

Stage-like thinking about both dying and grief has been appealing to many people. Somehow the "stages of grief" have helped people make sense out of an experience that isn't as orderly and predictable as we would like it to be. If only it were so simple! The concept of "stages" was popularized in 1969 with the publication of Elizabeth Kubler-Ross' landmark text On *Death and Dying.* Kubler-Ross never intended for people to literally interpret her five "stages of dying." However, many people have done just that, not only with the process of dying, but with the processes of bereavement, grief, and mourning as well. Often people around the grieving person believe that he or she should be in "stage 2" or "stage 4" by now. Nothing could be further from the truth. Each person's grief is uniquely his or her own. It is neither predictable nor orderly. Nor can its different dimensions be so easily categorized. We only get ourselves in trouble when we try to prescribe what the grief and mourning experiences of others should be-or when we try to fit our own grief into neat little boxes.

Myth #3: It is best to move away from grief and mourning instead of toward it.

Many grievers do not give themselves permission or receive permission from others to mourn. We live in a society that often encourages people to prematurely move away from their grief instead of toward it. Many people view grief as something to be overcome rather than experienced. The result is that many of us either grieve in isolation or attempt to run away from our grief. People who continue to express their grief outwardly-to mourn-are often viewed as "weak," "crazy" or "self-pitying." The common message is "shape up and get on with your life." Refusing to allow tears, suffering in silence, and "being strong," are thought to be admirable behaviors. Many people in grief have internalized society's message that mourning should be done quietly, quickly, and efficiently. Such messages encourage the repression of the griever's thoughts and feelings. The problem is that attempting to mask or move away from grief results in internal anxiety and confusion. With little, if any, social recognition of the normal pain of grief, people begin to think their thoughts and feelings are abnormal. They may say, "I think I'm going crazy!" They're not crazy, just grieving. And in order to heal they must move toward their grief through continued mourning, not away from it through repression and denial.

Myth # 4: Tears expressing grief are only a sign of weakness.

Unfortunately, many people associate tears of grief with personal inadequacy and weakness. Crying on the part of the mourner often generates feelings of helplessness in friends, family, and caregivers. Out of a wish to protect mourners from pain, friends and family may try to stop the tears. Comments such as, "Tears won't bring him back" and "He wouldn't want you to cry" discourage the expression of tears. Yet crying is nature's way of releasing internal tension in the body and allows the mourner to communicate a need to be comforted. Crying makes people feel better, emotionally and physically. Tears are not a sign of weakness. In fact, crying is an indication of the griever's willingness to do the "work of mourning."

Myth #5: The goal is to "get over" your grief.

We have all heard people ask, "Are you over it yet?" To think that we as human beings "get over" grief is ridiculous! We never "get over" our grief but instead become reconciled to it. We do not resolve or recover from our grief. These terms suggest a total return to "normalcy" and yet, the person is forever changed by the experience of grief. For the mourner to assume that life will be exactly as it was prior to the death is unrealistic and potentially damaging. Those people who think the goal is to "resolve" grief become destructive to the healing process. Mourners do, however, learn to reconcile their grief. They learn to integrate the new reality of moving forward in life without the physical presence of the person who has died. With reconciliation a renewed sense of energy and confidence, an ability to fully acknowledge the reality of the death, and the capacity to become re-involved with the activities of living. Acknowledging pain and grief are difficult-yet necessary-parts of life and living.

As the experience of reconciliation unfolds, the grieving person recognizes that life will be different without the presence of the person who died. At first this is realized in the mind, and later it is realized the heart. Reconciliation is a process, not an event. The sense of loss does not completely disappear yet softens and the intense pangs of grief become less frequent. Hope for a continued life emerges as commitments to the future are made. The person who died will never be forgotten, yet life can and will move forward.

Appendix B: Examples of Grief Rituals

- Buy a very special candle and light it at times that are special to your loved one's memory (e.g. birthday, Father's Day, anniversaries, etc.)

- Write special notes in balloons and let them go

- Feed the hungry/homeless at Thanksgiving, holidays, etc. in memory of the loved one

- Create a scrapbook of memories, photos

- Create ancestor rituals e.g. sprinkle rose petals around the pictures of deceased relatives as a part of other ceremonies e.g. weddings

- Plant a strong, healthy tree or rosebush in a loved one's name

- Create a memorial garden and add a new plant on an anniversary

- Find a tree and tie a yellow ribbon around it. Go there to remember. This is especially helpful when ashes have been scattered and there is no grave site.

- Offer a scholarship in a loved one's name

- On birthdays, holidays, anniversaries buy a gift in memory of your loved one and donate it to someone in need.

- At special religious times of year, bring out a special item in remembrance of your loved one

- Have wedding ring made into a new setting (e.g. a necklace, braclet etc.)

- Have a birthday celebration for your loved one and invite guests to wear the deceased's favourite colour and enjoy his or her favourite food.

- Have a family "memory" evening where you share pictures, reminisce about special times, or create a scrapbook of memories, etc.

Our lives are punctuated by before and after moments that shape our existence. Before the death of a loved one, we live in the reality that we later define as the world before the death. After the death, we live in another reality: the world after the death. They are literally two different worlds. Ritual does not harmonize these worlds, nor does it bridge the chasm between them. It does, however, open a temporary imaginative space where we begin to come to terms with the loss of the other world. So long as the wounds of loss need mending, the work of ritual will continue. Mourning rituals do not repair reality; they repair the survivor, but only partially. For the bereaved the world remains forever changed and forever broken: they do not magically heal from the "slings and arrows of outrageous fortune". And yet, through the ongoing, creative process of mourning, those wounded by loss can find hope, healing, and a way forward in their journeys in grief. (Scott, 2009)

Many religions and cultures have rituals that can be meaningful for those who are grieving regardless of their culture or religion. For an example of a Native American grief ritual see www.staurosusa. wordpress.com/2009/12/22/the-gifts-of-native-american-spirituality-and-grief-rituals-that-help/.

Appendix C: Supporting Children Through Dying and Death

1. Accept that it is not easy. You may:
   - Be upset and stressed
   - Be unable to concentrate
   - Lack energy
   - Want to protect your child from pain
   - Not know what the child understands
   - Be concerned about the effect of the death on the child

2. Be prepared for resistance from others. People may say:
   - They don't know what's going on
   - Wait until later
   - Make up a story
   - Don't say anything
   - Send them away until the funeral is over
   - Don't put them through this

3. Parents and family should know that children:
   - Read emotions around them
   - Respond to body language
   - Ask questions directly or indirectly
   - Remember that it is impossible not to communicate to children
   - Do not assume that a child who does not ask questions is not aware

4. Children should know:
   - Why you are sad
   - Why others are sad
   - Why they are sad
   - It is okay to be sad
   - The sadness was not caused by anything they did or didn't do

5. The grieving adolescent needs:
   - Parental support
   - Peer support
   - Caring/consistent home life
   - Freedom to express grief through open communication, ritual, music, dance, art
   - Time to trust

REACH OUT FOR HELP!

Chapter Eleven

Occupational Wellness

Thriving in Hospice Palliative and End-of-Life Care

Those who work in hospice palliative care are witness to and engage in an endless tide of illness, death and bereavement. Everyone is touched by involvement with the dying and bereaved and the impact leaves us with an appreciation of each and every day as well as a real awareness of the fragility of life. The challenge that caregivers have is to find a way to be emotionally involved in their work; to take their empathy, helping motivations, commitments and idealism and use them without succumbing to stress related illnesses.

What attracts staff to Hospice Palliative Care?

Vachon and Huggard (2010) note that a study conducted in New Zealand identified the following five themes related to choosing to work in the field of hospice palliative care.

- Previous death of a close family member that was an exceptionally good experience can lead to a desire to be part of something that provides exemplary support at a vulnerable time in people's lives. On the other hand, deaths that involve extreme pain or other unmanaged symptoms can lead to a desire to improve the care of the dying.

- Some may choose hospice palliative care as part of a career development path wanting to become more specialized in this particular field of practice.

- Some appreciate the work environment. e.g. are drawn to the holistic nature of the care and value being a member of an interdisciplinary team.

- Some are drawn to hospice palliative care because the values and philosophy espoused in hospice palliative care align with their personal values.

- Some choose hospice palliative care for personal lifestyle reasons e.g. spiritual calling, service to others, flexibility in hours, shifts, work close to home.

A number of studies cited in Vachon and Huggard (2010) offer insight into the practice of nurses and physicians in hospice palliative care. Georges and colleagues identified the following two methods of practice:

1. Striving to adopt a well-organized and purposeful approach which included the following:
   a. Using a scientific classification system (diagnosis and interventions)
   b. Working within the limits set by policy
   c. Developing a professional attitude: focusing on identified tasks, on the clarity and completeness of information sharing as opposed to the emotional impact of the message
   d. Striving to remain objective and consciously avoid allowing feelings to impact the response to situations
   e. Being task orientated and measuring outcomes of interventions
   f. Avoiding emotional stress by remaining professional and detached
   g. Embracing a practitioner-focused perspective which is characterized by a distant approach to patients and a well-developed self awareness to work on personal development as a professional

2. Striving to increase the well-being of the patient involved the following approaches:
   a. Using professional capabilities (e.g. being sensitive to the person's concerns) and adapting the approach to the individual
   b. Adopting a humble attitude in which personal considerations were put aside in an effort to show availability without expecting anything of the person in return
   c. Giving attention to the person and his or her experience as evidenced by efforts to discover and understand what the person is experiencing and the reason for particular reactions
   d. Sharing information based on the premise that adequate and complete information leads to informed decision making

   e. Being available or truly present and trusting intuition

   f. Valuing a caring attitude based on an authentic relationships with each person

   g. Remaining attentive and thoughtful and adopting a person centered attitude

   h. Trying to accept and cope with emotional strain as part of the reality instead of avoiding the strain; remaining authentic even if problems could not be fully alleviated

Another study, Huggard proposes that comfort in working with the dying is preceded by a growth and development process which involves the following stages of adaptation: (Vachon & Huggard, 2010)

1. Intellectualization

2. Emotional survival

3. Depression

4. Emotional arrival

5. Deep compassion

6. The Doer

In order to become the "Doer" and practice the art as well as the science, mentors are invaluable.

Occupational Stressors

A stressor is any experience that disrupts homeostasis. Positive stressors are rewarding or adaptive while negative stressors are harmful and threatening yet frequently are the impetus that prompts change. Ongoing negative stressors can contribute to stress related illnesses.

Stressors arise from both internal and external sources. Internal stressors are linked to balancing home responsibilities with work life, self expectations and struggling with the continuous formation and loss of relationships. External stressors are linked to inadequate training or support to deal with the cumulative impact of death and grief, conflict in the workplace, or discrepancies in the values beliefs and goals within the care team. The discrepancy between one's vision of good hospice palliative care and the reality of the care provided at the bedside can be a major cause of distress. (Thompson and Wainwright 2006)

Some of the distressing issues that formal caregivers involved in the current health system contend with include:

- Lack of respect from other team members
- Team conflict
- Ruthless obstinacy, aggressive treatment when burden outweighs benefit
- Demanding consumers
- Lack of physicians, nurses and other caregivers
  - Aging of the workforce
- Experienced clinicians reaching retirement age
- Increasing costs
- Inadequate resources
- Increasing accountability
- Job insecurity

- Aging of the population
  - Increasing numbers of geriatric patients
  - Increasing numbers of patients with cancer and other progressive life limiting illnesses
- New treatments that lead to living longer with chronic illness
- Increased complexity of care and treatment related to a person having more than one chronic illness
- Shift to community based care from traditional institution based care

Vachon and Huggard (2010) present a model for understanding occupational stress. The framework includes six areas of worklife.

1. Workload

   Excessive workload exhausts the health care provider and emotional work is especially draining when the job requires the individual to display emotion inconsistent with feelings. Current issues with the nursing shortage, and fiscal restraint all have an impact on worklife.

2. Control

   Control is related to insufficient control over the resources necessary to do the work or insufficient authority to pursue the work in what is believed to be the most effective manner. Lack of communication skills and / or management skills and expectations to assume responsibility with inadequate training can lead to difficulty in functioning. Other issues of control can involve safety, the timing of referrals, feeling responsible for symptom management when the person with authority to address the issue is unresponsive to the need, and emotional involvement without sufficient supervision or support.

3. Rewards

   Salary or benefits that are not commensurate with achievements or lack of social rewards when work is not appreciated by others can lead to dissatisfaction. Intrinsic rewards e.g. doing something of importance and doing it well can counterbalance the mismatch.

4. Community

   When team members are ordered about without consultation or participation, they will not give their best efforts. Conflict among staff members contributes to emotional exhaustion and depersonalization. Manageable shifts, informal support from peers, adequate orientation, management of staff conflict and feedback that acknowledges that you are doing a good job have been reported as valued initiatives.

5. Fairness

   Fairness communicates respect, confirms self worth and in the work environment may be the tipping point between engagement or burnout. Rivalries between staff and programs as well as unfair reimbursement systems continue to be issues.

6. Values

   Being able to work in an area in which values are consistent with personal values aids in job satisfaction. Respondents in the study talked of the sense of purpose and the sacredness of the work, making a difference, loving the job and passion for what I do; all indictors of how meaningful and rewarding hospice palliative care can be.

How health care providers involved in hospice palliative care respond to the stressors in their work lives will vary according to personal, professional and environmental differences. Factors that affect response include:

- Level of training in dealing with dying, death and grief
- Organizational support and commitment .e.g. designated time for collaborative work, opportunity for team review and evaluation, flexibility and openness to new ideas
- Team support e.g. access to expertise, respect for the skills of each team member, synergy and camaraderie
- Communication and conflict resolution
- Life experiences
- Personality
- Coping strategies

When distress is overwhelming and coping mechanisms are ineffective the health care provider can succumb to one of the stress related syndromes. There are many names given to the syndromes that result from workplace distress e.g. compassion fatigue, moral distress, burnout, vicarious trauma, or battle fatigue.

- **Compassion Fatigue** is a danger for all those in the helping professions. Symptoms include having no energy, feeling empty, having nothing left to give, feeling depleted in every dimension, and having too many questions and no answers (Wright, 2004). Compassion fatigue symptoms are closely related to those of post traumatic stress disorder but it applies to those who are emotionally affected by trauma to another. (Vachon and Huggard, 2010)

- **Moral Distress** occurs when various options for action are available but there are competing and not easily reconciled values and beliefs of right and wrong underlying the choices. Having to act contrary to personal or professional values undermines authenticity and integrity. (Wasylenko 2011)

- **Burnout** is a consequence of being stressed over a protracted period of time. Burnout impairs the quality of the social environment at work and is seen as the final step in a progression of unsuccessful attempts to cope with a variety of negative stress conditions (Vachon and Muller 2009).

- **Vicarious Trauma** is the process of change that happens due to caring about other people who have been hurt, and feel committed or responsible to help them. Over time this process can lead to changes in psychological, physical, and spiritual well-being. (Headington Institute 2011)

- **Battle Fatigue** is a term that originated in WW II and today would be called post traumatic stress disorder. The person with PTSD is typically numb with symptoms of depression, excessive irritability, survivor guilt, recurrent nightmares, flashback to the traumatic scene, and overreaction to sudden noises.

Compassion fatigue and burnout share similar characteristics but those suffering from compassion fatigue are able to continue caring (Vachon and Muller 2009). Re-emergence is possible; the despair and sense of hopelessness can be addressed if caregivers are open to each other's care and concerns.

Symptoms of stress related illness are listed in the table below.

Symptoms of stress related illness.
(Figley, 2002)

Cognitive	Emotional	Behavioural	Spiritual	Personal Relations	Somatic	Work Performance
Lowered concentration	Powerlessness	Impatient	Questioning the meaning of life	Withdrawal	Shock	Low morale
Decreased self esteem	Anxiety	Irritable	Loss of purpose	Decreased interest in intimacy or sex	Sweating	Low motivation
Apathy	Guilt	Withdrawn	Lack of self satisfaction	Mistrust	Rapid heartbeat	Avoiding tasks
Rigidity	Anger/rage	Moody	Pervasive hopelessness	Isolation from others	Breathing difficulties	Obsession about details
Disorientation	Survivor guilt	Regression	Anger at God	Overprotection as a parent	Aches and pains	Apathy
Perfectionism	Shutdown	Sleep disturbances	Questioning prior religious beliefs	Protection of anger or blame	Negativity	Lack of appreciation
Minimization	Numbness	Nightmares	Loss of faith in a higher power	Intolerance	Dizziness	Detachment
Preoccupation with trauma	Fear	Appetite changes	Greater scepticism about religion	Loneliness	Increased number and intensity of medical maladies	Poor work commitments
Thoughts of self harm or harm to others	Helplessness	Hyper vigilance		Increased interpersonal conflicts	Other somatic complaints	Staff conflicts
	Sadness	Elevated startle response			Impaired immune system	Absenteeism
	Depression	Accident proneness				Exhaustion
	Emotional roller coaster	Losing things				Irritability
	Depleted					Withdrawal from colleagues
	Overly sensitive					

Job engagement which is the opposite of burnout involves energy, involvement and effectiveness; it is characterized by high levels of activity and pleasure. Schaufeli and Bakker (2004) define engagement as a positive, fulfilling, work-related state of mind that is characterized by vigour, dedication, and absorption. Vigour is characterized by high levels of energy and mental resilience while working, the willingness to invest effort in one's work, and persistence also in the face of difficulties. Dedication is characterized by a sense of significance, enthusiasm, inspiration, pride, and challenge. Absorption is characterized by being fully concentrated and happily engrossed in one's work, whereby time passes quickly and one has difficulties with detaching oneself from work. Maintaining job engagement requires a sustainable workload, feelings of choice and control, appropriate recognition and reward, a supportive work community, fairness and justice, as well as meaningful and valued work.

There are many factors that contribute to the personal and/or team distress of those working in the current health care system. While organizations have some responsibility for ensuring job satisfaction and competency, health care providers are also accountable for their own personal and professional well-being. Each team member can benefit from learning how to constructively deal with issues and conflicts. Incorporating proven stress management techniques into daily life will benefit both the individual and the team as a whole.

Vachon and Huggard (2010) identify personal, professional and organizational responsibilities for health care professionals working in hospice palliative care.

Personal

- Self care questionnaire
- Self care contract
- Work-Life-Balance
- Restorative activities
- Time with family and friends
- Stress management
- Exercise and nutrition
- "Learn to say no"
- Assertiveness
- Accept help and support
- Fun
- Next holiday planned and booked
- Nurturing, caring and valuing self
- Spiritual and religious needs

Professional

- Collegial Support
- Reflective practice
- Professional development
- Effective Communication
- Maintain motivation
- Prioritize workload
- Manage time
- Taking meal breaks
- Humour
- Attend to grief work

Organizational

- Recruitment and orientation
- Accurate job descriptions
- Competencies linked to performance appraisals
- Human Resources Policies and Procedures
- Training opportunities – Support for study
- Communication channels
- Critical Incident Debriefing
- Regular feedback
- Healthy roasters
- Acknowledgement of personal pressures
- Staff support

The Palliative Care Community

- Develop and maintain networks
- Local
- Regional
- Provincial
- National
- International

A sense of commitment, control and pleasure in one's work have been identified as primary personal coping mechanisms. (Vachon and Haggard 2010). Other characteristics identified by researchers in the field of stress include a sense of coherence (a feeling of confidence that one's life is orderly, manageable and meaningful), a sense of congruence (a feeling of rapport within oneself, a sense that the internal and external aspects of one's being are in agreement with one another), as well as the personality construct of hardiness.

Hardiness

Dr. Susan Kobasa conducted research in the stress hardiness field in the 1970s. Commitment, control and challenge are the characteristics of hardiness. (IB Psychology 2011)

- **Commitment:** The hardy individual is one who is involved with life and life's activities such as work, family, and friendships.

- **Control:** The hardy individual has a sense of control over things that happen in his or her work and personal life.

- **Challenge:** The hardy individual tends to see a challenge where others may perceive a threat.

Cognitive hardiness has been a predictor of the ability to manage job stress, anxiety, daily hassles and to maintain a healthy lifestyle. Cognitive hardiness refers to a specific set of attitudes or beliefs about work and life that are relatively enduring from day-to-day. A sense of commitment and strong interest toward work, family, hobbies, or projects that you are involved in on a day-to-day basis as well as having things that you look forward to doing are indications of cognitive hardiness. A sense of belonging with friends, work, and family are other components of cognitive hardiness. When cognitive hardiness is present, daily life changes are seen as being challenging rather than threatening. Change affords hidden opportunities for new experiences and growth as opposed to being a hindrance to work and life satisfaction. The belief that you have control over your life, that what you do is directly related to what you achieve, and that success in work and life is a result of individual behavior rather than luck, fate, or chance supports cognitive hardiness. A belief that you can effectively achieve success in both work and life appears to buffer the potentially damaging impact of stress on well-being and directly generates effective coping behaviours.

Stamm (2002) notes that those with more time to sustain relationships and basic self-care tasks seem to be less at risk for experiencing the negative effects of caregiving. See Appendix A for basic self care ideas.

Resilience is another means of preventing, minimizing or overcoming the damaging effects of adversity. Resilience is the product of a complex relationship of specific psychological inner strengths and environmental social supports throughout a person's life that determines the response to adversity. Resiliency springs from within and is also integrated with the quality of relationships and positive experiences that help people of all ages acquire hope, motivation, mastery, values and a sense of purpose (Resiliency Institute 2011). Developing resiliency is now recognized as a vitally important requirement for the health and well-being of everyone. The promotion of resilience lies in "encountering stress at a time and in a way that allows self confidence and social competence to increase through mastery and appropriate responsibility" (Vachon and Huggard 2010). See Appendix B for aspects of resiliency.

Caring does not come without cost. Experiencing the fear, pain and suffering of others has an impact on caregivers. The most effective therapists are the most vulnerable because of their enormous capacity for feeling and expressing empathy. True service is not a relationship between an expert and a problem; it is far more genuine than that. True service is a relationship between people who bring the full resources of their combined humanity to the table and share them generously (Remen, 2000).

Hospice palliative care requires a balancing act. Caregivers need to grieve. Those who do not grieve losses are at risk; however, caregivers cannot allow their hearts to become so filled with loss that they have no room left to care.

Caregivers want to experience compassion satisfaction; a sense of efficacy and happiness. When caregiver efforts are making the world in which they live a reflection of what they believe it should be, they experience fulfillment and live a life that is characterized by enthusiasm, dedication, energy, involvement, and effectiveness.

It is important for caregivers to remember to care for themselves so that they can care for others. They are encouraged to create a community of care rather than feeling solely responsible for meeting the needs of others; to connect to whatever is personally meaningful and be playful and attentive to the "spirit" at work (Medland, Howard-Ruben, & Whitaker 2004).

Perhaps real wisdom lies in not seeking answers at all. Any answer we find will not be true for long. An answer is where we fall asleep as life moves past us to the next question. After all these years I have begun to wonder if the secret of living well is not in having all the answers but in pursuing unanswerable questions in good company.

Rachael Naomi Remen (2000)

Reference List

Figley, C. (2002). *Treating compassion fatigue*. New York: Brunner-Routledge.

Headington Institute. (2011) *Understanding and addressing vicarious trauma*. Retrieved from www. headington-institute.org/Default.aspx?tabid=2648

IB Psychology. (2011) *Hardiness: Kobasas Key Study*. Retrieved from http://ibpsychology.wetpaint. com/page/Hardiness%3A+Kobasas+Key+Study May 2011.

Medland, J., Howard-Ruben, J., & Whitaker, E. (2004). Fostering psychosocial wellness in oncology nurses: addressing burnout and social support in the workplace. *Oncology nursing forum*. 31(1):47-54.

Remen, R.N. (2000). *My grandfathers blessings*. New York: Riverhead Books.

Resiliency Institute. (2011) *What is Resiliency?* Retrieved from http://www.resiliencyinstitute.com/ resiliencyInformation/whatIsResiliency.php April 2011

Schaufeli,W. &, Bakker, A. (2004). Job demands, job resources, and their relationship with burnout and engagement: a multi sample study. Journal of Organizational Behaviour 25, 293-315. Published on line in Wiley InterScience (www.interscience.wiley.com)

Siebert, A. (2006) *How to Develop Resiliency Strengths*. Retrieved from www.resiliencycenter.com/ articles/survresiliency.shtml April 2011

Stamm, B. (2002). Measuring compassion satisfaction as well as fatigue: developmental history of the compassion satisfaction and fatigue test. In C. Figley (Ed.) *Treating compassion fatigue*. New York: Brunner-Routledge.

Thompson, M. & Wainwright, W. *Stressors and Self-care for Professionals* (2006) In *Medical Care of the Dying*. Victoria Hospice Society Learning Centre for Palliative Care.

Vachon, M. & Huggard, J. (2010). The Experience of the Nurse in End-of-Liffe Care in the 21st Century: Mentoring the Next Generation. In B.R. Ferrell & N. Coyle (Eds.) *Textbook of Palliative Nursing*. (Chapter 61). New York: Oxford University Press.

Vachon, M & Muller, M. (2009). Burnout and Symptoms of Stress in Staff Working in Palliative Care. In H.M.Chochinov & W. Breitbart (Eds.) *Handbook of Psychiatry in Palliative Medicine*. New York: Oxford University Press.

Wright, B. (2004). Compassion fatigue: how to avoid it. *Palliative Medicine*. 18:1, 3-4.

Wasylenko, E. (2011) *Addressing Moral Distress in Caregiving at End of Life*. Retrieved from www. ualberta.ca/~bioethic/Health%20Ethics%20Week/AddressingMoralDistressingatEndofLife.pdf

Appendix A: Self Care Ideas

1. Diversion
   - Spend time alone. See a movie. Daydream.
   - Write. Paint. Create something. Try scrapbooking.
   - Take a class. Read. Join a club.
   - Play an instrument. Sing. Listen to music.
   - Play a game. Go out with friends.
   - Tackle a new project. Keep busy. Volunteer.

2. Family
   - Balance time at work and home. Accept the good with the bad.
   - Look for win/win solutions.
   - Build good family feelings. Focus on strengths. Take on new family roles. Stay open to change.
   - Develop friendships with other families. Make use of community resources
   - Take time to be together. Build family traditions. Express affection.

3. Interpersonal
   - Believe in yourself. Trust others. Give compliments.
   - State your needs and wants. Say "no" respectfully.
   - Make new friends. Really listen to others. Touch if appropriate.
   - Show feelings. Share feelings.
   - Accept others' boundaries. Drop some involvements.
   - Share problems with others. Ask for support from others.

4. Mental
   - Look for the humour. Anticipate the future.
   - Set clear goals. Plan for the future.
   - Take charge. Make order. Don't let things pile up.
   - Solve it yourself. Seek outside help. Tackle problems head-on.
   - Change perspective. Look for good in a bad situation.
   - Focus on top priorities. Work smarter, not harder.

5. Physical
   - Listen to your body. Know your physical limitations.
   - Pursue physical fitness. Jog. Swim. Dance. Walk.
   - Take short stretch breaks throughout your day.
   - Eat for health. Limit use of alcohol.
   - Tense and relax each muscle. Take a warm bath. Breathe deeply.
   - Energize your work and play. Strive for self-improvement.

6. Spiritual
   - Take up a worthy cause. Invest yourself meaningfully.
   - Find purpose and meaning. Share beliefs with others.
   - Confess. Ask forgiveness. Pray for others. Give thanks.
   - Let go of problems. Learn to live with the situation.
   - Set priorities. Be consistent. Spend time and energy wisely.

Appendix B: Developing Resiliency

Adapted from *How to Develop Resiliency Strengths* by Al Siebert, Ph.D., author of *The Resiliency Advantage*

Develop a playful, childlike curiosity. Ask lots of questions, want to know how things work. Play with new developments. Enjoy yourself as children do. Have a good time almost anywhere. Wonder about things, experiment, make mistakes, get hurt, laugh. Ask: "What is different now? What if I did this? Who can answer my questions? What is funny about this?"

Constantly learn from experience. Rapidly assimilate new or unexpected experiences and facilitate being changed by them. Ask "What is the lesson here? What early clues did I ignore? The next time that happens I will...."

Adapt quickly. Be mentally and emotionally flexible. Be comfortable with contradictory personality qualities. Be both strong and gentle, sensitive and tough, logical and intuitive, calm and emotional, serious and playful; the more the better. Think in negative ways only to reach positive outcomes e.g. "What could go wrong, so it can be avoided?"

Have solid self-esteem and self-confidence. Self-esteem determines how much you learn after something goes wrong. It allows you to receive praise and compliments. It acts as a buffer against hurtful statements while being receptive to constructive criticism. "I like, appreciate, and love myself...."

Be self-confident; it is your reputation with yourself. Self confidence allows you to take risks without waiting for approval or reassurance from others. You expect to handle new situations well because of your past successes. "These are my reliable strengths...."

Have good friendships, loving relationships. Research shows that people in toxic working conditions are more stress resistant and are less likely to get sick when they have a loving family and good friendships. Loners are more vulnerable to distressing conditions. Talking with friends and family diminishes the impact of difficulties and increases feelings of self-worth and self-confidence.

Express feelings honestly. Experience and express anger, love, dislike, appreciation, grief--the entire range of human emotions honestly and openly. Choose to suppress feelings when you believe it would be best to do so.

Expect things to work out well. Be optimistic guided by internal values and standards. Have a high tolerance for ambiguity and uncertainty. Working without a job description is a good model of professionalism. Expecting things to work out well has a synergistic effect, it brings stability to crises and chaos. Ask "How can I interact with this so that things turn out well for all of us?"

Read others with empathy. See things through the perspectives of others, even antagonists. Develop a win/win attitude when conflicts arise. Ask "What do others think and feel? What is it like to be them? How do they experience me? What is legitimate about what they feel, say, and do?"

Use intuition, creative hunches. Accept subliminal perception and intuition as valid, useful sources of information. Ask "What is my body telling me? Did that daydream mean anything? Why don't I believe what I'm being told? What if I did this?"

Defend yourself well. Avoid and block attacks, fight back. See through and side-step cons, "games," and manipulations that others attempt. Find allies, resources, and support.

Have a talent for serendipity. Learning lessons in the school of life is the antidote to feeling victimized. Convert a situation that is emotionally toxic for others into something emotionally nutritious for them. Learn good lessons from bad experiences; convert misfortune into good luck and gain strength from adversity. A good indicator of exceptional mental health is when a person talking about a rough experience says "I would never willingly go through anything like that again, but it was the one of best things that ever happened to me." Ask "How can I turn this around? Why is it good that this happened? What is the gift?"

Get better and better every decade. Become increasingly life competent, resilient, durable, playful, and free. Enjoy life more and more.

Chapter Twelve

Definitions

Definitions: Commonly Used Terms

Reference: Ferris, F.D., Balfour, H.M., Bowen, K., Farley, J., Hardwick, M., Lamontagne, C., Lundy, M., Syme, A., & West, P. (2002). *A model to guide hospice palliative care; Based on national principles and norms of practice.* Ottawa: Canadian Hospice Palliative Care Association.

Activities of daily living

Daily personal care activities, including ambulation, bathing, toileting, feeding, dressing and transfers. May also include cooking, cleaning, laundry, banking, shopping.

Advance directives

A person's formal or informal instructions concerning expectations of care and choice of treatment options in response to potential illnesses or conditions (legal connotations vary by jurisdiction; includes a living will).

Accountability

The fiduciary and professional responsibility to those receiving care and the community.

Alternate, complementary, integrative therapies

Terms often used to describe independent healing systems outside the realm of conventional medical theory and practice.

Assess

To identify, describe, evaluate and validate information.

Autonomy

The state of being self-governed.

Beneficence

The provision of benefits and the balancing of harms and benefits for the purpose of doing the most good.

Care

All interventions, treatments and assistance to the person and family.

Care plan

See "Plan of Care"

Caregiver

Anyone who provides care.

Formal caregivers are members of an organization and accountable to defined norms of conduct and practice. They may be professionals, support workers, or volunteers. They are sometimes called "providers."

Informal caregivers are not members of an organization. They have no formal training, and are not accountable to standards or conduct or practice. They may be family members or friends.

Confidentiality

The protection and control of information privy to persons.

Discrimination / prejudice

Any act by another that inhibits a person's ability to fully participate in society, especially when related to age, gender, national and ethnic origin, geographical location, race, colour, language, creed, religion, sexual orientation, diagnosis, disability, availability of a primary caregiver, ability to pay, criminal conviction, family status.

Essential services

The critical services required to implement the plan of care.

Essential step

Any activity that is required to meet a stated objective.

Expectations

Issues, hopes, and fears identified by the person and / or family that require attention in the plan of care.

Family

Those closest to the person in knowledge, care and affection.

> May include:
- the biological family
- the family of acquisition (related by marriage / contract)
- the family of choice and friends (including pets).

The person defines who will be involved in his or her care and / or present at the bedside.

Goal

> A desired future condition:
- statement of intent
- broader in focus than an objective
- specific enough to indicate direction and thrust
- quantitative or qualitative.

Grief

Sorrow experienced in anticipation of, during and after a loss.

Hospice palliative care

Care that aims to relieve suffering and improve the quality of living and dying

Illness

Absence of wellness due to disease, another condition, or aging.

An **acute illness** is one that is recent in onset and likely to be time-limited. If severe, it could be life threatening.

A **chronic illness** is likely to persist for months to years. With progression it may become life threatening.

An **advance illness** is likely to be progressive and life threatening.

A **life-threatening illness** is likely to lead to death in the near future.

Interdisciplinary care team (related to person / family care)

A team of caregivers who work together to develop and implement a plan of care. Membership varies depending on the services required to address the identified issues, expectations, needs and opportunities. An interdisciplinary team typically includes one or more physicians, nurses, social workers/psychologists, spiritual advisors, pharmacists, personal support workers, and volunteers. Other disciplines may be part of the team if resources permit.

Justice

The fair treatment of all individuals, without discrimination or prejudice.

Life closure

The process of putting personal, social (including financial and legal), and spiritual affairs in order, giving of gifts (e.g. personal treasures, money, etc), creation of a legacy, reminiscence, and saying goodbye in preparation for death. This usually occurs close to the end of a person's life.

Measure

To find out the extent, size, quantity, capacity, etc.

Mission

A short statement of an organization's purpose; what it is and what it does.

Needs

Issues identified by caregivers that require attention in the plan of care.

Nonmaleficence

The avoidance of doing harm.

Norm

A statement of usual or average practice. Less rigid than a standard.

Objective

A desired accomplishment or hoped for result:
- specific
- narrower in focus than a goal (may flow from a goal and be a means to achieve a goal)
- quantitative and measurable.

Outcome

A measurable end result or consequence of a specific action or essential step.

Pain

An individual, subjective, unpleasant sensory and emotional experience that is primarily associated with tissue damage or described in terms of tissue damage, or both.

Patient

The person living with an acute, chronic, or advanced illness.

The term **patient,** as opposed to **client,** is used in recognition of the individual's potential vulnerability at any time during the illness. The word **patient** derives from the Latin *patiens:* to suffer, to undergo, to bear.

The patient is a contributing member of the interdisciplinary team.

Plan of care

The overall approach to the assessment, management, and outcome measurement to address the expectations and needs prioritized as important by the person and family.

Policy

A course of action selected from alternatives and in light of given conditions to guide and determine present and future decisions.

Preferred practice guideline

The recommended approach to guide the provision of care related to a particular issue. Must be flexible to take into account the exceptions/variations needed to meet the wide range of person/family expectations and needs. May be consensus or evidence based.

Principle

A fundamental truth.

Provider

A formal caregiver who is a member of an organization and accountable to defined norms of conduct and practice. The may be professionals, support workers, or volunteers.

Program

An organization with a number of component parts. It may be part of a larger host organization, or independent. It may or may not have its own governance structure.

Proxy

A person or agency of substitute recognized by law to act for, and in the best interest of the person.

Quality care

The continuous striving by an interdisciplinary team/program to meet the expectations and needs of the persons and families it serves.

Quality of life

Well-being as defined by each individual.

It relates both to experiences that are meaningful and valuable to the individual, and his/her capacity to have such experiences.

Regional team

Regional teams are functional units within hospice palliative care organizations designed to provide formal caregivers and oversight to multiple patients/family care teams within a given population/region/setting of care.

Risk

A measure of the presence of variables that are likely to contribute to the development of an undesirable illness or condition.

Setting of care

The location where care is provided.

Settings for hospice palliative care may include the person's home, and acute, chronic, or long-term care facility, a nursing home/skilled nursing facility, a hospice or palliative care unit or freestanding facility, a jail or prison, the street, etc.

Service

An organization providing assistance or service to others. Services tend to be part of a larger organization (e.g., a host organization or a program). They have one or more component activities. Most will not have their own governance structure.

Spirituality

An existential construct inclusive of all the ways in which a person makes meaning and organizes his/her sense of self around a personal set of beliefs, values and relationships.

This is sometimes understood in terms of transcendence or inspiration. Involvement in a community of faith and practice may or may not be a part of an individual's spirituality.

Standard

An established measurable condition or state used as a basis for comparison for quality and quantity.

Strategies

The specific methods, processes, or steps used to accomplish goals and objectives. Strategies impact resources (inputs) in some positive or negative way. They are executed in a tactical manner so as to link goals and objectives to day-to-day operations.

Suffering

A state of distress associated with events that threaten the intactness of a person. It may be accompanied by a perceived lack of options for coping.

Tactics

The specific actions that link goals to day-to-day operations.

Therapeutic relationship

A relationship between skilled caregivers and the person/family that aims to change the person's and family's experience of illness and bereavement. It combines the art and science of the process of providing care with the knowledge and skills needed to deliver a wide range of therapeutic interventions.

Total pain

Suffering related to, and the result of, the person's physical, psychological, social, spiritual and practical state.

Truth-telling

The communication of what is known or believed to be true without deceit or falseness. Persons may voluntarily decline to receive information and designate someone else to receive information on their behalf, as long as there is no evidence of coercion.

Unit of care

Those who are the focus of a plan of care. In hospice palliative care this is typically the person and his/her family.

Value

A fundamental belief on which practice is based.

Vision

A short statement of an organization's aspirations; what it hopes to become and achieve.

Volunteer

A person who freely gives of his/her time, talent, and energy.

Volunteers are members of an organization and accountable to that organization's standards of conduct and practice.